Symptoms, Signs and

A Medical Glossary

CW00358118

Other Books of Interest

Abbreviations in Medicine
E. B. Steen, PhD

Baillière's Midwives' Dictionary
Vera da Cruz SRN, SCM, MTD
Margaret Adams SRN, SCM, MTD, DN

Baillière's Nurses' Dictionary
Barbara F. Cape SRN, SCM, DN(Lond)
Pamela Dobson SRN, SCM, RNT

Baillière's Pocket Book of Ward Information
Marjorie Houghton OBE, SRN, SCM, DN(Lond)
L. Ann Jee SRN, Part I CMB, RNT

Symptoms, Signs and Syndromes
A Medical Glossary

B. CHAMPNEY SRN, RNT
*District Nursing Officer, Western District, Leeds AHA (Teaching);
formerly Director of Nurse Education, School of Nursing, General
Infirmary, Leeds*

F. G. SMIDDY MD, ChM, FRCS
*Consultant Surgeon, General Infirmary, Leeds, and Clayton Hospital,
Wakefield; Senior Clinical Lecturer, University of Leeds; formerly
Senior Lecturer, Professorial Surgical Unit, Leeds*

BAILLIÈRE TINDALL · LONDON

A BAILLIÈRE TINDALL book published by
Cassell Ltd,
35 Red Lion Square, London WC1R 4SG
and at Sydney, Auckland, Toronto, Johannesburg
an affiliate of
Macmillan Publishing Co. Inc.
New York

© *1979 Baillière Tindall*
a division of Cassell Ltd

All rights reserved. No part of this publication may be reproduced,
stored in a retrieval system or transmitted in any form or by any
means, electronic, mechanical, photocopying or otherwise, without the
prior permission of Baillière Tindall, 35 Red Lion Square, London
WC1R 4SG

First published 1979

ISBN 0 7020 0712 9

Printed in Great Britain by
Butler & Tanner Ltd, Frome and London

British Library Cataloguing in Publication Data

Champney, B
  Symptoms, signs and syndromes.
  1. Semiology 2. Nursing
  I. Title II. Smiddy, Francis Geoffrey
  616.07′2′024613   RT65

  ISBN 0–7020–0712–9

Preface

The symptoms of a disease and the physical manifestations (or signs) of the underlying pathological process are the starting points for the diagnosis of the majority of illnesses. It is the authors' strong belief that the professions ancillary to medicine, nurses and physiotherapists in particular, are provided by their close and enduring contact with patients in the ward with an invaluable opportunity to observe the changing pattern of human disease.

With this in mind we have chosen to describe those symptoms and signs and their underlying physio-pathological causes, where these are known, which are the manifestations of the commoner diseases.

It has long been medical custom that when a number of symptoms and signs occur together a name is given to them (commonly the name of the physician who first saw the association); this association is called a syndrome.

The choice of subject matter no doubt reflects our own interests; we hope these interests will be shared by the reader.

We would like to thank Mrs P. Docherty, Mrs K. Simpson and Miss M. Dunwell without whose unremitting labour this glossary could not have been produced.

August 1978   BETTY CHAMPNEY
                                       GEOFFREY SMIDDY

How to use this glossary

The entries are arranged in alphabetical order, as in an ordinary dictionary. Each entry starts with a definition of the term, followed by an explanation, if this is known, of the particular phenomenon and a description of its characteristic features.

The reader may be unfamiliar with some of the terms used in the explanations. For ease of cross-reference, those terms printed in capital letters have their own full entry at the appropriate point in the glossary.

Abdominal pain

Abdominal pain is a symptom of many conditions. It may be acute or chronic, constant or intermittent, continuous or colicky and it may or may not be associated with readily recognizable signs of peritoneal irritation.

(1) Conditions within the abdomen giving rise to abdominal pain include:
  (a) Diseases of hollow organs, e.g. duodenal ulceration, chronic cholelithiasis, strangulation, or virus infections such as mesenteric adenitis.
  (b) Diseases involving the peritoneum including chemical or bacterial peritonitis.
  (c) Vascular conditions such as mesenteric arterial or venous thrombosis, or dissecting aneurysm.
  (d) Sudden 'distension' of the capsule of the liver as in right sided heart failure.
(2) Conditions outside the abdomen giving rise to abdominal pain:
  (a) REFERRED PAIN, originating in the heart, diaphragm or chest wall.
  (b) Metabolic causes of pain in which the mechanism by which abdominal pain is produced is not entirely clear, including diabetic KETOSIS, PORPHYRIA, URAEMIA.
  (c) Toxic causes including lead poisoning.
(3) Neurogenic pain caused by diseases of the spinal cord or nerve roots, e.g. spinal cord tumours or virus infections such as herpes.
(4) Psychogenic pain of which one of the most classical is MUNCHAUSEN'S SYNDROME.

Abdominal swelling

Generalized abdominal swelling is usually a sign of:
(1) An accumulation of abdominal fat.
(2) Gas in the intestinal tract.
(3) Fluid in the peritoneal cavity—ASCITES.
(4) Faeces in the colon.
(5) Pregnancy, giant ovarian cysts or massive fibroids.

The symptom, in contrast to the actual presence of abdominal swelling, is not uncommon in neurotic patients who will often complain of a sensation of tightness requiring the loosening of constricting clothing.

(1) Fat. Abdominal swelling due to adipose tissue is usually part of a generalized OBESITY. Rarely is it a sign of the hormonal derangement produced by CUSHING's disease or syndrome in which abnormal quantities of adreno-cortical hormones are secreted. In this condition excessive fat normally accumulates on the trunk and proximal parts of the limbs.

(2) Gas accumulates in the intestinal tract in excessive quantities in the presence of mechanical or paralytic obstruction. The former is normally associated with vomiting and intestinal COLIC whereas the latter may be relatively painless despite the gross abdominal distension which occurs.

(3) ASCITES. The accumulation of excessive quantities of fluid in the peritoneal cavity which must be distinguished from the swelling produced by a large ovarian cyst or occasionally a full bladder.

(4) Faeces. An excess of faeces sufficient to cause generalized abdominal distension is rare. It may, however, occur in 2 conditions.

   (a) Hirschsprung's disease, a congenital condition in which the parasympathetic nerve supply to the rectum and possibly the colon is absent so that the bowel fails to empty. In the majority of affected babies this condition becomes evident soon after birth when the abdominal distension becomes obvious and the baby fails to pass meconium.

   (b) Idiopathic megacolon, a condition in which there is no demonstrable anatomical abnormality of the bowel. This disorder begins usually at 3 to 4 years of age and is believed to be caused by some psychological upset during potty training.

(5) The presence of a fetus. The generalized abdominal swelling caused by full-term pregnancy may be

mimicked by the presence of large fibroids of the uterus although the presence of a fetal heart beat serves to distinguish between the two conditions.

Abscess

A collection of pus in a cavity lined by granulation tissue. Clinically abscesses of bacterial origin are often described as 'hot' when caused by pyogenic bacteria and 'cold' when caused by infection with organisms such as the *Mycobacterium tuberculosis*. The former are associated with fever, the overlying skin is redder and warmer than its surroundings and the abscess is painful. A 'cold' abscess causes none of these symptoms and if the overlying skin is affected at all it is cold to the touch and often bluish in colour. Either type may 'point' on a skin or epithelial surface whereupon the 'hot' abscess discharges its contents onto the surface and is usually cured, whereas a 'cold' abscess usually forms a SINUS.

The pus of a 'hot' abscess consists of bacteria, living and dead, dead tissue cells, polymorphonuclear leucocytes, proteolytic enzymes and a variety of chemical antibacterial substances including antibodies. The pus of a 'cold' abscess is described as caseous or cheesy because it is thicker and creamy yellow in colour. It contains living and dead mycobacteria, many lymphocytes and a fluid content rich in fat.

Whilst the majority of abscesses are caused by bacterial infection, non-bacterial agents such as chemicals are occasionally responsible. This type of abscess is normally sterile but may become infected to become a typical 'hot' abscess.

Acetonuria

The presence of acetone in the urine. The commonest cause of acetonuria is a lack of the hormone insulin. The result is a decrease in the rate of breakdown of glucose which is normally used by the tissues as their main source of energy. When this occurs the body begins to use fat and protein to provide its energy supply but in the absence of sufficient insulin these compounds are incompletely broken down. The result is the production of chemical substances known as ketone bodies, one of which is acetone. Of greater physiological importance is the production also of acetoacetic acid which when present in excessive quantities in the bloodstream causes ACIDOSIS. The presence of acetone and/or acetoacetic acid in the urine can be detected by the use of 'Acetest' tablets.

Acetone also appears in the urine in starvation when there is no disturbance of insulin secretion. This is again due to the body tissues having to use substances other than glucose to maintain the energy requirements of the body.

Achlorhydria

The absence of hydrochloric acid from the gastric juice caused by the disappearance of the acid-secreting parietal cells from the mucosal lining of the stomach. Achlorhydria occurs in pernicious anaemia even when potent stimulating agents such as histamine or pentagastrin are used. It is also common in patients suffering from cancer of the stomach, but unlike pernicious anaemia, the administration of histamine or pentagastrin still causes the production of acid.

Acholuric jaundice

A type of JAUNDICE in which the skin and tissues become yellow but there is no increase in the amount of bile pigment in the urine which therefore remains of normal colour.

The underlying cause of this type of jaundice is always an excessive destruction of erythrocytes which leads to the release into the circulation of increasing quantities of haemoglobin from which the bile pigments are formed. Should the quantity formed be greater than the liver cells can excrete, jaundice occurs. The urine, however, remains a normal colour because unconjugated bile pigment, that is pigment which has not passed through a liver cell, is insoluble in water and therefore cannot be excreted in the urine by the kidney.

Excessive erythrocyte destruction (haemolysis) occurs in:

(1) Conditions associated with alterations in shape of the erythrocyte. The classical example of this is hereditary spherocytosis in which the red cells are no longer biconcave but spherical. This alteration in shape causes these cells to be more fragile than normal and they are there-

fore broken down more easily and after a shorter time in the circulation than are normal erythrocytes.

(2) Conditions associated with alterations in the chemical composition of haemoglobin such as sickle cell anaemia in which the red cells twist and alter in shape and are destroyed when exposed to low oxygen tensions.

(3) Exposure of the erythrocytes to antibodies. If anti-erythrocyte antibodies are present in the circulation, the red cells are haemolysed, as after a mis-matched blood transfusion.

(4) Miscellaneous causes of excessive haemolysis include thermal burns in which the red cells are destroyed by heat and SEPTICAEMIA in which the red cells are destroyed by the various bacterial toxins.

In acholuric jaundice the stools and the urine remain normal in colour because there is no obstruction to the flow of bile pigment from the liver into the duodenum. When the condition is chronic as in hereditary spherocytosis, stones composed of bile pigment are finally deposited in the gall bladder. In the course of time these may later cause obstructive jaundice.

Acidosis

An increase in the acidity of the blood, the chemical reaction of which is normally kept constant by regulatory mechanisms involving the lungs and the kidneys.

The symptoms of acidosis include:

(1) DYSPNOEA due to stimulation of the respiratory centre in the brain stem by the increasing acidity of the blood. Increased depth and rate of respiration blows off carbon dioxide and, therefore, tends to lower the concentration of carbonic acid in the blood.

(2) Mental confusion and loss of consciousness occur when the condition becomes serious, hence the COMA of uncontrolled diabetes.

(3) Since many of the causes of acidosis are also associated with abnormal levels of circulating potassium, cardiac irregularities including CARDIAC ARREST are not uncommon.

The causes of acidosis are commonly divided into two:

(1) Respiratory acidosis which occurs in patients suffering from severe pulmonary disease such as chronic bronchitis in which carbon dioxide cannot be eliminated from the lungs. The gas remaining in the circulation forms carbonic acid.

(2) Metabolic acidosis which may be caused by:

    (a) The excessive production of acidic materials in the body as in the condition of diabetic KETOSIS.

    (b) Severe renal damage in which the kidneys are unable to excrete the acidic materials formed during normal metabolic processes. It is this latter type of acidosis which is complicated by a rise in the concentration of potassium in the blood to levels which are incompatible with normal cardiac function.

    (c) An excessive loss of alkaline substances from the body as a result of severe DIARRHOEA or from small intestinal FISTULAE.

Acromegaly

A sign of over-secretion of growth hormone by the anterior lobe of the hypophysis cerebri after fusion of the epiphyses has occurred. Compare this to GIGANTISM. An excess of this hormone results in generalized hyperplasia of the tissues with the result that the bones of the extremities, jaw and face enlarge, producing the characteristic features of the acromegalic which include prominent ridges above the eyes, a protruding lower jaw and enlargement of the hands. The disease is associated with osteoporosis which results in loss of strength in the bones so that the vertebral bodies collapse and a KYPHOSIS develops. Loss of libido and diabetes mellitus are also common.

Agranulocytosis

The disappearance of the polymorphonuclear white blood cells from the circulation, often accompanied by a pancytopenia in which all the cellular elements of the blood, i.e. erythrocytes and platelets also disappear. The condition should be suspected when a patient suddenly develops a reduced resistance to infection. This occurs because the disappearance of the granulocytes removes one of the main defences of the body against bacterial invasion. Commonly severe fever and ulceration of the gums, oral mucosa and throat occur, later followed by fungal infection.

The diagnosis is easily made by full blood count, differential white count and an examination of the bone marrow.

Among the many causes of agranulocytosis are the toxic effects of many therapeutic agents including:

(1) Phenylbutazone, used in the treatment of arthritis.
(2) Thiouracil, used in the treatment of thyrotoxicosis.
(3) Chloramphenicol, used in the treatment of bacterial infections.
    With these drugs there is seldom a relationship between the amount of the drug which has been received and the occurence of agranulocytosis.
(4) The alkylating agents such as thiotepa used in the treatment of malignant disease. The incidence and severity of the agranulocytosis following the administration of these drugs is related to the dose.

Albinism

Albinism is a sign of an inherited enzyme deficiency. Although pigment cells are present in normal numbers, the pigments which normally colour the skin and eyes cannot be produced due to absence of one specific enzyme known as tyrosinase. The result is an individual with a pale skin, white hair and pink eyes. Albinos are rare, occurring 1 in 10 to 20 000 births.

Albright's syndrome

A syndrome, the cause of which is unknown, associated with marked deformity of the skeleton, precocious puberty in girls and skin pigmentation. During the growing period prior to closure of the epiphyses, bone is replaced by dense fibrous tissue which is a poor substitute. The bones in this condition are then incapable of supporting the body and the weight-bearing bones bend leading to severe bowing of the lower limbs.

Albuminuria see PROTEINURIA

Aldrich's syndrome

A hereditary disorder transmitted by a sex-linked gene which affects only boys in whom PURPURA, THROMBOCYTOPENIA, eczema and recurrent skin infections occur. The possible cause is a failure of IMMUNITY to develop.

Alkalosis

A condition in which the blood is more alkaline than normal—that is the pH is raised above the normal value of 7.4.

Alkalosis is either metabolic or respiratory:

(1) Metabolic alkalosis occurs when there is an excess of alkali in the blood brought about by:
   (a) The ingestion of excessive quantities of alkali, usually the result of the treatment of duodenal ULCERATION. In this case the patient may develop NAUSEA, VOMITING and ANOREXIA.
   (b) The loss of acid from the body by excessive vomiting or gastric aspiration as the gastric juice contains hydrochloric acid. Alkalosis due to this cause is nearly always associated with the signs of DEHYDRATION and TETANY, with the development of a positive CHVOSTEK'S SIGN.

(2) Respiratory alkalosis is caused by any condition which produces a persistent increase in the depth and rate of respiration (hyperventilation). This leads to the excessive extraction of carbon dioxide from the blood in the lungs which produces a fall in the level of carbonic acid in the blood. Respiratory alkalosis is common in hysteria and at high altitudes when respiration is stimulated by the lack of oxygen.

The principal result of alkalosis of respiratory orgin is to precipitate the onset of TETANY, even though the serum calcium level remains normal.

Alkaptonuria

The presence in the urine of homogentisic acid. If such urine is allowed to stand it turns brown or black in colour. The presence of such a pigment is due to an error in protein metabolism. The condition is rare and is inherited through a recessive gene. Normally there is no evidence of the condition until middle age when about this time a breakdown product of homogentisic acid begins to be deposited in the sclerotics of the eye. Deposition of the same pigment in cartilage, tendons and ligaments leads to darkening of the cheeks and nose and ARTHRITIS.

Allergy

A sign of an altered reaction by the tissues to antigens which, in this particular case, are known as allergens.

There may be a subtle difference between ALLERGY and ANA-PHYLAXIS (hypersensitivity) since the latter implies an excessive reaction to an antigen, but most authorities use the two terms synonymously. Two types of allergy are recognized, the distinction being made according to the speed with which the reaction begins. In the first type, the reaction occurs almost immediately, whereas in the second it is delayed for 24 to 48 hours.

The immediate type of reaction is due to interaction between the allergen and antibodies already circulating in the blood stream, whereas in the delayed type the reaction is the result of a reaction between the allergen and the cells of the tissue.

Colloquially, the term allergy is applied to the reaction which follows the inhalation of pollen or dust, the eating of certain foodstuffs such as shellfish or strawberries, contact with plants such as the primula, or materials such as furs, and the response to the administration of certain drugs, for example, penicillin. The reaction varies—when the allergen is inhaled, rhinitis, hay fever or asthma occur; skin contact produces URTICARIA and the injection of an allergen may produce a generalized anaphylactic reaction resulting in death.

Amblyopia

Blurring of vision. In childhood amblyopia is usually caused by difficulty in fusing the separate visual images which pass to the brain from the eyes. To overcome this difficulty, the image from one eye is suppressed in order to prevent DIPLOPIA (double vision), but as a result visual perception is reduced.

9

Later, because of the disuse following suppression, the visual pathway deteriorates. Amblyopia of one eye may also occur if there is a high refractive error.

In an adult, amblyopia may be caused by a number of conditions affecting the cells of the retina or the optic nerve. These include disseminated sclerosis, which damages the nerve and poisons such as quinine, methylated spirits and tobacco, which damage the retina. Amblyopia may also be a symptom of HYSTERIA.

Amenorrhoea

Absence of menstruation is divided into two types.

(1) False amenorrhoea in which menstruation is taking place, but the outflow is obstructed, for example by an imperforate hymen.

(2) True amenorrhoea which may be divided into physiological and pathological varieties:

(a) The physiological types occur:

(i) Prior to puberty and during adolescence due to the absence of hormonal stimulation.

(ii) In pregnancy, amenorrhoea occurs due to the continuous production of large quantities of the hormones oestrogen and progesterone by the chorion.

(iii) During lactation, when amenorrhoea results from lack of formation of the hormones known as gonadotrophins.

(iv) During the menopause, when the ovaries cease to react to the gonadotrophic stimulus.

(b) Pathological types. Since the maintenance of the menstrual cycle depends on the proper functioning of the hypothalamus, the anterior lobe of the pituitary gland, the ovary and the uterus, any disturbance of this chain may result in amenorrhoea.

Amenorrhoea is, therefore, observed in FROHLICH'S SYNDROME, in conditions causing injury or disease of the midbrain such as encephalitis or meningitis, and in cerebral conditions such as depressive illnesses. Disease of the pituitary, usually in the form of destructive conditions which reduce or eliminate the gonadotrophic hormones, also causes amenorrhoea, thus SHEE-HAN'S (SIMMOND'S) SYNDROME in which necrosis of the anterior pituitary gland follows childbirth, is always accompanied by amenorrhoea. Ovarian amenorrhoea follows the under-production of oestrogen and progesterone as in the Stein Leventhal syndrome in which the ovaries are slightly enlarged and polycystic.

Amnesia (Loss of memory)

Amnesia only occurs when the mechanisms associated with the ability to memorize break down. Before a memory can be established, attention must be directed to the retention of the idea or event with which the individual is concerned. If, therefore, the mind is diverted or preoccupied an event may occur which fails to register in the mind. This may occur in perfectly normal individuals when it is referred to as 'absent minded-ness', but is more commonly seen in patients suffering from severe ANXIETY.

Memory also depends upon the integrity of certain portions of the brain which are particularly concerned with this activity. These are mainly those parts of the cerebral cortex known as the parieto-occipital region, the temporal lobe and a much deeper part of the brain known as the hippocampus.

Common conditions leading to amnesia include:

(1) Head injuries. Blows on the head may produce a state of unconsciousness lasting for minutes, hours or days. When consciousness returns there is usually a period of loss of memory for events prior to the accident known as retrograde amnesia and a period following the accident known as post-traumatic amnesia. In assessing the severity of the brain injury the post-traumatic amnesia is more important than the retrograde. Following recovery from the injury the memory may be impaired and, although great improvement usually occurs over a period of several months, if full recovery has not occurred within 2 to 3 years, a permanent defect can be expected.

(2) Epilepsy. Amnesia always occurs during an epileptic

attack. If the patient suffers from petit mal the period of amnesia may be so transitory as to be of little importance. However, in grand mal the period of amnesia may persist for an hour or more.

(3) ANXIETY and HYSTERIA may both be associated with amnesia. The former is often associated with inattentiveness and therefore a reduced capacity to memorize an event, whilst in the latter a complete amnesia for past events is not uncommon.

Anaemia

A sign rather than a disease. The underlying cause must always be identified and, if possible, corrected.

The term implies a fall in the amount of haemoglobin in the blood, which may be due either to a decrease in the amount of pigment in each erythrocyte or to a decrease in the number of erythrocytes. Normally these number 4.5 to 6.5 million/mm³ in the male and somewhat less in the female.

In fetal life the cells of the blood, i.e. erythrocytes, granulocytes and platelets, are produced in all parts of the reticuloendothelial system including the liver and spleen, but in the last 3 months of intrauterine life the marrow gradually predominates in the production of blood cells. In the adult the red marrow in which erythropoiesis occurs is restricted to the cancellous tissue at the ends of long bones, the membranous bones and the vertebrae. In conditions in which an increased production is required the red marrow extends.

In order to produce a normal red cell the bone marrow requires an adequate supply of various building materials including protein, vitamins, iron and copper. Not only must a person ingest an adequate diet, he must also be able to absorb them from the intestinal tract.

In addition the endocrine glands of the body must be normal. Deficiency of adrenal, thyroid or pituitary hormones all lead to anaemia.

The common causes of anaemia are:

(1) Excessive bleeding in which the red blood cells are usually normochromic. The loss of blood may be obvious, e.g. a wound, HAEMATEMESIS, EPISTAXIS or it may be con-

cealed as in a ruptured ectopic gestation. Chronic blood loss leading to severe anaemia is common in disorders of menstruation, haemorrhoids or new growths affecting the gastrointestinal tract.

(2) Defective red cell production which usually occurs when one of the building materials necessary for haemopoiesis is diminished resulting in:

    (a) Iron deficiency anaemia in which the red cells apart from being diminished in numbers are also deficient in the amount of pigment which they contain.

    (b) Vitamin B_{12} deficiency which may be the result of:

        (i) Deficiency of the gastric intrinsic factor such as occurs in pernicious anaemia.

        (ii) Diseases of the lower part of the small bowel such as Crohn's disease which lead to defective absorption.

        (iii) Abnormal growth of bacteria in the small bowel, which assimilate the vitamin for their own metabolism thus reducing the amount available to be absorbed. This is the cause of anaemia following the development of strictures or blind loops in the small bowel.

    Vitamin B_{12} deficiency is accompanied by a macrocytic anaemia in which the erythrocytes are larger than normal.

    (c) Folic acid deficiency which may result from:

        (i) Dietary deficiency.

        (ii) Impaired absorption by the small bowel.

        (iii) Increased requirements as in pregnancy.

(3) Excessive red cell destruction, the haemolytic anaemias. These are divisible into two main groups.

    (a) Hereditary, in which there is either an abnormality in the structure of the red cell as in congenital spherocytosis or an abnormality of the haemoglobin molecule as in thalassaemia.

    (b) Acquired, in which the basic abnormality lies outside the erythrocytes themselves.

(i) The destruction may be the result of antibodies, see KERNICTERUS.

(ii) Bacterial, metabolic, or chemical toxins, as in SEPTICAEMIA, URAEMIA or lead poisoning.

Anaphylaxis and the anaphylactic reaction

A type of reaction which may be caused by the interaction of an antigen with antibody, such a reaction causing local or general effects. Examples of local reactions are asthma, hay fever and certain forms of contact dermatitis. In asthma and hay fever the antigen, usually dust, pollen or insect fragments, is inspired and reacts with antibody which has already been formed as the result of previous exposure to the antigen. This reaction occurs in the lung tissue causing the release of chemical substances such as histamine and serotonin. These in turn cause the muscle coat around the smaller air passages (bronchioles) to contract, producing bronchospasm and great difficulty in breathing.

A general reaction known as anaphylactic shock, is accompanied by acute respiratory distress, gross OEDEMA causing swelling of the eyelids and dependent parts, oedema of the larynx, which may add to the distress already caused by the bronchospasm, itching, a fall in blood pressure and even death. A general reaction of this type, which is also caused by the liberation of histamine, may follow repeated injections of horse serum, e.g. A.T.S. (Anti-Tetanus Serum), bee stings or occasionally after drugs such as penicillin. Some protection from an anaphylactic reaction can be produced in the human by a process known as desensitization. Once it is established that an individual is sensitive to a particular antigen, increasing doses are administered, commencing with amounts which are too small to provoke a reaction. This causes the production of such excessive quantities of antibody that the action of the antigen is blocked if future exposure occurs. Desensitization is commonly used in the treatment of patients suffering from hay fever and asthma.

Angina

A term which is most commonly used to describe the symptoms

produced by cardiac ischaemia. Less commonly to indicate the presence of a severe infection of the mouth and throat.

The main symptom of angina of cardiac origin is a severe crushing pain in the chest, sometimes radiating down the arm and up into the neck. This is frequently precipitated by exercise when the condition is known as angina of effort or by emotional stress such as anger or excitement. The pain is immediately relieved by rest or the relaxation of emotional tension. The development of angina indicates that the supply of oxygenated blood to the heart muscle (myocardium) is inadequate when the heart increases its work load by contracting more strongly and more rapidly as in exercise or in response to emotional excitement.

The commonest cause of such inadequacy is narrowing of the coronary arteries by atherosclerosis but occasionally severe anaemia leads to the same effect due to the reduced oxygen-carrying capacity of the blood.

The pain of angina is probably caused by stimulation of the sympathetic nerve endings in the myocardium. These reach the heart from the upper 4 or 5 segments of the spinal cord, at which level the spinal nerves carrying impulses from the skin of the chest and arms also reach the cord. When stimuli arise from the heart the brain interprets them as coming from the chest and arms, hence, so far as the patient is concerned, angina is a pain arising in these areas of the body. This type of pain, felt in one part of the body and brought about by disease in another, in this case the heart, is known as REFFERRED PAIN.

Angio-neurotic oedema

A term used to describe an ANAPHYLACTIC REACTION which produces severe OEDEMA of the face, hands and feet and, less commonly, the larynx. Laryngeal oedema is particularly serious, because it may cause death from asphyxia.

The commonest cause of angio-neurotic oedema is the sudden development of sensitivity to some article of diet, such as sea-foods, eggs or strawberries, less commonly to a drug such as penicillin.

15

Angio-neurotic oedema is really a type of URTICARIA and untreated the swelling usually persists for about 48 hours.

Ankylosis

A sign indicating that the range of movement of a joint has diminished. Ankylosis is usually classified as true or false.

A true ankylosis is caused by conditions such as tuberculous or pyogenic infections which destroy the joint surfaces themselves. As recovery from such infection occurs the bone ends are usually joined together by fibrous tissue or bone. A fibrous ankylosis obviously permits some movement of the joint whereas bony union causes complete fixation.

A false ankylosis is caused by conditions affecting structures outside the joint itself, such as tendons, muscles, fascial layers or skin. A relatively common example of a false ankylosis is Dupuytren's contracture, in which the fascia on the palmar surface of the hand slowly thickens and contracts leading to an ever increasing flexion deformity of the fingers. If this condition remains untreated, a secondary shortening of the joint capsules of the affected fingers follows, so that even when the diseased fascia is totally removed, movement of the fingers remains restricted.

Anorexia

Lack of appetite. In a normal individual the appetite is very delicately controlled so that despite the large amounts of food which may be eaten the body weight may change only slowly. Experimental evidence in the animal and physical disease in the human suggests that the major centre controlling appetite is in that part of the brain known as the hypothalamus. Damage to different parts of this area of the brain may result in either loss of appetite or alternatively a voracious appetite associated with increasing OBESITY.

Anorexia is, therefore, a common symptom of neurological or psychological disorders. It is extremely common in depressive illnesses or anxiety and an extreme form of appetite loss may occur in the condition known as anorexia nervosa. This condition is most common in adolescent girls and may result in a complete refusal to take food and end in death.

Anorexia also occurs if the stomach itself is the site of disease. Chronic alcoholics commonly lose their appetite due to the inflammation of the gastric mucosa which occurs and in carcinoma of the stomach anorexia is one of the commonest symptoms.

Fever and general malaise are also commonly associated with anorexia which disappears as soon as the patient's general feeling of well-being returns.

Anosmia

A loss of smell. This sensation is transmitted from the sensory area in the upper third of the nasal cavities to the brain by means of the olfactory nerves.

The common causes of anosmia include:

(1) Obstruction of the nasal passages which prevents inspired air reaching the sensory area in the nose. This is commonly due to polyps, but may be caused by a blood clot following a head injury.

(2) Lesions of the olfactory nerve itself which are most commonly caused by head injuries severe enough to cause fractures of the cribriform plate through which the nerve fibres pass on their way from the nose itself to the interior of the cranium. It may also be caused by inflammatory lesions affecting the base of the brain such as tuberculous meningitis or tumours arising in the brain which destroy the nerve pathways.

Anoxia

A lack of oxygen in the tissues. In clinical practice the degree of tissue anoxia is usually measured by estimating the oxygen pressure in the blood.

The basic causes of anoxia are:

(1) Anoxaemic anoxia: In this type the pressure of oxygen in the alveoli of the lung is reduced due either to a decreased oxygen pressure in the atmospheric oxygen or to inadequate breathing. This, the commonest form of anoxia, occurs in pulmonary diseases such as chronic

bronchitis or pneumonia and in individuals living at high altitudes.

(2) Anaemic anoxia: ANAEMIA from any cause leads to a diminished capacity of the blood to carry oxygen.

(3) Stagnant anoxia: An inadequate supply of oxygen to the tissues may occur if the circulation in the arterioles and capillaries is severely disturbed. This type of anoxia is frequently encountered in severe SHOCK caused by certain Gram-negative bacterial toxins because the muscular walls of the small blood vessels in the peripheral circulation are paralysed and the endothelial lining is destroyed causing the blood to stagnate in the affected vessels.

(4) Histotoxic anoxia: The ability of tissue cells themselves to use oxygen may be destroyed by disturbances of cellular enzymes. An example of this type of anoxia is cyanide poisoning.

The symptoms and signs associated with anoxia depend upon the rapidity of its onset and its severity. When it is acute, adaptation to the altered circumstances may be impossible and the first symptoms, as in a mountain climber, may be a decrease in vision, an increase in the respiration rate and TACHYCARDIA. This is followed by faulty mental judgement and later still, unconsciousness and death. When chronic anoxia occurs, as in persons living for long periods at high altitude, compensation is achieved by increasing the rate and depth of respiration and the oxygen-carrying capacity of the blood by the production of greater numbers of erythrocytes. A similar polycythaemia also occurs in patients suffering from chronic pulmonary disease in order to compensate in part for their reduced respiratory capacity.

Anuria

Urine is not formed by the kidney. The causes of this are:

(1) The blood flow through the kidney is so reduced, as in SHOCK, that glomerular filtration ceases and therefore no urine is formed. This is known as pre-renal anuria and if the condition is reversed prior to the development of

18

organic damage to the kidney, normal urine formation will begin again.

(2) The actual kidney is damaged—renal anuria. This may be caused by:

(a) Natural diseases such as glomerulo-nephritis and congenital cystic disease,

(b) It may follow severe shock which has not been adequately treated. This causes damage either to the glomeruli, a condition known as cortical necrosis, or damage to the renal tubules. Cortical necrosis is irreversible and can only be treated by intermittent dialysis or renal transplantation. Damage to the renal tubules, variously known as tubular necrosis or lower nephron nephrosis is usually reversible, although the patient may require dialysing for a limited period.

(c) Poisons: lead, phosphorus, the sulphonamides and some antibiotics such as kanomycin will damage the kidney.

(3) The outflow of urine from the kidneys is blocked. This is commonly caused by obstruction to the outflow of urine from the bladder by enlargement of the prostate, but occasionally it may follow the impaction of a stone in the ureter of a solitary kidney.

Whatever the underlying cause, untreated anuria leads to URAEMIA.

Anxiety

An emotion which is normally felt by most individuals in response to a dangerous situation and which may be associated with bodily disturbances such as PALPITATIONS, choking, overbreathing, TREMOR or DIARRHOEA. A normal person may have little sense of fear when anxious, but considerable bodily disturbance. An individual's reaction is abnormal only when anxiety is disproportional to the apparent danger.

Occasionally pathological anxiety is precipitated by an organic illness, such as HYPERTHYROIDISM but more often it is produced by some 'upsetting' event such as the loss of a close relative, the loss of a job or the prospect of an operation.

Acute anxiety may become panic, but more often a patient lives in a state of continual anxiety to which adaptation occurs. When, however, adaptation does not occur the patient's ability to enjoy living may be entirely destroyed.

Aphasia

A sign of damage to the central nervous system in which understanding of the written or spoken word or speech is affected, the particular disability depending on the area of the brain which has been destroyed.

Damage to the left cerebral hemisphere (in a right-handed person) produces an inability to understand either the spoken or written word—sensory aphasia. Alternatively a patient may be able to comprehend what is said, or even recognize an object, but is unable to speak—motor aphasia. The presence of aphasia localizes the damage done to the brain, usually by injury, tumours, thrombosis of supplying blood vessels or degeneration, to the area of the cortex.

Other types of aphasia which occur include agraphia when a patient is unable to express himself in writing, this occurs when the parietal lobes are damaged. Agnosia, when a patient is unable to recognize the nature or use of a familiar object, indicates destruction of the temporal lobes.

Aphonia

Loss of voice. Aphonia may be due to FUNCTIONAL or organic causes.

(1) Functional aphonia usually occurs in young women who are subjected to undue stress. The voice may be lost completely or more commonly reduced to a whisper. Sudden recovery may occur. Examination of the larynx shows that the cords do not come together (adduct) on phonation but do so on COUGHING.

(2) Organic aphonia is caused by:

    (a) Local diseases of the larynx such as INFLAMMATION or cancer.

    (b) Interruption of the nerve supply to the muscles of the larynx. The motor nerves to the larynx are the recurrent laryngeal nerves and these may be damaged at any point from their origin in the brain to their entry into the larynx. Common causes of such damage include:

   (i) Vascular accidents in the brain, i.e. a STROKE.
  (ii) Tumours of the neck, e.g. malignant thyroid tumours.
 (iii) Accidental injury as in the operation of thyroidectomy.

Apnoea

A sign that respiration has ceased.

Respiration is normally controlled by a number of nerve cells arising in the base of the brain which are collectively known as the respiratory centre; through its effect on the intercostal and phrenic nerves this centre initiates the contraction of intercostal muscles and diaphragm and so of inspiration.

The respiratory centre is especially sensitive to the concentration of carbon dioxide in the blood. Should this be reduced, e.g. by taking a series of rapid, deep breaths, the respiratory centre is no longer stimulated and a period of apnoea follows. During this interval carbon dioxide once again accumulates in the blood and, on reaching a critical level, respiration recommences.

Any lesion causing damage to the respiratory centre may result in apnoea, hypoxia and death. In the newborn, interference with the placental circulation either at the placenta itself, or by pressure on the cord, may lead to brain damage due to fetal asphyxia. In an adult the respiratory centre may be damaged by a severe head injury, although this is nearly always a secondary effect due to the increasing intracranial pressure which produces coning. A commoner cause is the temporary cessation of respiration leading to CHEYNE–STOKES RESPIRATION which is seen in HEART FAILURE.

Apraxia

Clumsy or awkward movements occurring in patients who are not actually paralysed due to a disturbance of motor activity.

21

The cause of apraxia is a disturbance of either the frontal or parietal cortex of the brain in which the idea and formulation of movements are constructed.

When the frontal cortex is damaged ideomotor apraxia develops in which the patient is unable to plan a particular movement and therefore appears clumsy. If the parietal cortex is damaged the patient is unable to carry out a planned action because he cannot build up in his mind a correct pattern of movement. This is known as ideational apraxia and it produces bizarre performances such as trying to strike a cigarette on a matchbox in order to light a match held in the mouth.

Argyll Robertson pupil

A pupil which does not constrict (become smaller) on exposure to a bright light, but which constricts when accommodating, i.e. focusing on a near object.

The common cause of this type of pupil is damage to a small group of nerve cells known as the ciliary ganglion, sometimes by injury and occasionally by bacterial infections such as syphilis.

Arthritis

A term which literally means INFLAMMATION of a joint, but in one of the commonest forms of joint disease, osteoarthrosis (osteoarthritis), inflammation plays no part at all.

Although no underlying disease is present in the majority of patients suffering from arthritis, in a minority some general cause can be identified. Secondary or symptomatic arthritis occurs in:

(1) Metabolic disorders such as gout in which characteristically the first metatarso-phalangeal joint becomes inflamed and arthritic due to deposition of urate crystals in the cartilage of the joints and the surrounding soft tissues. Acute gouty arthritis is often accompanied by severe pain and tenderness in the joint, together with redness of the overlying skin.

(2) Blood disorders such as HAEMOPHILIA in which the joint is destroyed by repetitive haemorrhages into the joint

space. The resulting haemarthrosis is organized by invasion with granulation tissue.

(3) Neurological disorders such as syphilis in which proprioceptive sensation disappears from the soft tissues around the joint with the result that the joint and its capsule are exposed to excessive stresses and strains.

(4) Gastrointestinal disorders such as ulcerative colitis. In this condition a 'rheumatoid-like' type of arthritis is not uncommon.

Ascites

A condition in which free fluid accumulates within the peritoneal cavity. Ascites is a symptom and sign of:

(1) Malignant cells deposited on the lining of the peritoneum. These cells multiply and produce a sterile exudate with a high protein content. When the exudate is examined microscopically, malignant cells recognized by their irregular size, shape and large dark-staining nuclei, are usually found in the fluid.

(2) Right-sided HEART FAILURE in which ascites is formed in the following way. As the muscles of the right side of the heart fail in strength, they are no longer able to pump blood through the lungs. In consequence, blood is dammed back from the right ventricle via the right atrium into the inferior and superior venae cavae. The increasing venous pressure in the inferior vena cava leads to congestion of the lower limbs which swell and become OEDEMATOUS. In addition, because blood from the liver and intestines eventually finds its way into the inferior vena cava, these organs are also engorged. This produces a rise in the pressure of blood in the hepatic circulation with the result that PORTAL HYPERTENSION develops. This causes a transudate from the surface of the liver. Any condition causing improper filling or emptying of the heart may lead to ascites.

(3) Cirrhosis. Three factors contribute to the formation of ascites in this condition:

(a) The portal venous pressure increases because structural changes in the liver produce venous obstruction and, therefore, portal hypertension, so that a transudate occurs from the surface of the liver.

(b) As the function of the liver cells diminishes they cease to manufacture albumin, one of the main proteins of the plasma, with the result that the protein concentration in the plasma falls. This reduces the osmotic pressure of the blood causing a loss of fluid from the circulation into the surrounding tissues.

(c) An excessive secretion of the adrenal hormone, aldosterone, occurs leading to a retention of sodium and water in the body and consequently OEDEMA.

(4) Hypoproteinaemia which may be caused by a variety of conditions including:

(a) Loss of protein in excessive quantities, e.g. in the urine in certain types of kidney disease, or via the intestinal tract if this is inflamed.

(b) Starvation, e.g. kwashiorkor.

(c) Extensive surgical resection of the bowel leading to inadequate absorption of protein.

(5) Inflammatory ascites. Ascites due to exudation of fluid into the peritoneal cavity occurs in chronic inflammatory conditions of the peritoneum such as tuberculosis.

Astigmatism

A sign associated with an abnormal curvature of the cornea and, to a lesser degree, of the lens. The resulting symptom is a blurring of the visual image due in part to the primary cause and partly because compensatory efforts are made by the muscles of the eye to focus the distorted image on the retina. These efforts often result in 'eye-strain' and HEADACHES.

Ataxia

Unsteady or clumsy movements due to loss of the normal smooth action. It is a sign of disease of the cerebellum and its connections, disorders of the labyrinths or loss of proprioception.

If the affected individual has difficulty in standing with the eyes open or staggers on turning, cerebellar or labyrinthine disturbance is most likely but similar symptoms may occur with proprioceptive loss. However, if only the latter system is involved the unsteadiness only becomes apparent with the eyes closed leading to a positive ROMBERG'S SIGN.

Cerebellar ataxia should be considered if the patient is unable to stand with the eyes open and when an intention tremor is present. This can be demonstrated by asking the patient to grasp an object. In attempting to do so the patient's fingers and hand persistently overshoot or undershoot the object and because they have not found their target are brought back and forth in further repeated attempts to conform to the order. Similarly in the legs attempts at the heel–knee test end in the same manner. Such signs of cerebellar ataxia are often associated with NYSTAGMUS and scanning speech.

The causes of cerebellar disturbance include:

(1) Congenital conditions such as Friedreich's ataxia in which the descending fibres from the cerebellum degenerate.
(2) Birth injury.
(3) Infarction, HAEMORRHAGE or tumours lying in or near the cerebellum.

Labyrinthine ataxia occurs as a result of diseases of the inner ear and its central connections. The onset may be rapid and associated with VERTIGO, TINNITUS and DEAFNESS. Repeated attacks of this type occur in Ménière's disease. Sensory ataxia is caused by proprioceptive loss from muscles, joints and tendons and is characteristically seen in tabes dorsalis or extensive peripheral neuropathies. The inco-ordination caused by loss of the afferent impulses is partially compensated for by using the eyes. This type of ataxia is commonly accompanied by loss of deep sensitivity and vibration sense.

Atelectasis

Strictly, this term means that a part or the whole of a lung has failed to expand at birth. If the lung has been inflated and has contained air in the alveoli and these, for some reason, become airless, the correct term to use is 'collapse'. However, these two terms are often used rather loosely.

Used in the correct sense the commonest cause of atelectasis is hyaline membrane disease which is caused by the cells lining the alveoli failing to secrete a chemical substance necessary to allow the alveoli to expand as inspiration begins. In the absence of this chemical known as a surfactant the bronchioles and alveoli remain atelectatic and death may occur within a few days.

Hyaline membrane disease occurs most commonly in premature infants weighing between 1 and 2 kg. Under the microscope individual alveoli cannot be distinguished because there has never been air in them. If the infant survives for more than a few hours, a protein membrane develops, which gives the disease its name, in the unaerated bronchioles.

The degree of respiratory difficulty caused is proportional to its severity from the moment of birth. The baby may be CYANOSED, because blood continues to flow through the affected parts of the lung but does not come in contact with oxygen because the alveoli are airless. When very severe, the chest wall is sucked in on inspiration because the atelectatic lung does not expand.

Athetosis

Intermittent attacks of increased tone in the voluntary muscles producing writhing movements or peculiar postures caused by a disorder of the central nervous system. A common characteristic is extreme hypertension of the fingers at the metacarpophalangeal joints.

The precise physiological explanation of athetosis is unknown. It is possibly caused by a disorder in the brain affecting nerve fibres passing from the cerebral cortex via the thalamus to the spinal cord. Athetoid movements are characteristic of children suffering from cerebral palsy due to perinatal cerebral ANOXIA, birth injury or KERNICTERUS.

Atrial fibrillation

A rapid and irregular contraction of the wall of the atria of the heart sometimes reaching 400 to 600 per minute which may be appreciated by the individual as persistent PALPITATIONS or the affected person may be completely unaware of the irregularity.

Atrial fibrillation is a sign of organic disease of the heart although it is sometimes caused by anaesthetic agents. The common conditions which may be followed by atrial fibrillation are rheumatic heart disease, ischaemic changes in the myocardium due to atherosclerosis of the coronary arteries and myocarditis. Fibrillation also may occur in thyrotoxicosis.

The rapid and unco-ordinated contractions of the atrial muscle cause:

(1) Incomplete emptying of the atria which in turn leads to incomplete filling of the ventricles and hence to a decreased cardiac output.

(2) Bombardment of the atrio-ventricular node which governs the rate of ventricular contraction with a large number of abnormal stimuli. The ventricular contractions become irregular at a rate usually varying between 100 and 150 per minute since the node cannot pass the majority of impulses through to the conducting system of the ventricle. Many of the irregular contractions are so weak that they do not eject sufficient blood from the heart to produce a palpable peripheral pulse in the radial artery at the wrist with the result that the pulse becomes irregular both in rhythm and volume. The difference between the countable apex beat and the radial pulse is known as the pulse deficit.

Atrial flutter

A rapid but regular contraction of the wall of the atrium due to a single abnormal focus of stimulation in its wall, the rate of discharge and hence the rate of contraction reaching 260 to 360 per minute. Flutter is invariably associated with organic heart disease including rheumatic, HYPERTHYROID or ischaemic disease.

The stimuli from the atria reach the atrio-ventricular node and the majority are impeded so that the eventual rate of ventricular contraction is only once for every 2, 3, or 4 atrial contractions.

Whereas in ATRIAL FIBRILLATION the ventricular beat and hence the radial pulse is irregular, in flutter the pulse usually remains regular but rapid. For this reason a patient may be aware of fibrillation and completely unaware of flutter.

Atrophy

A diminution in the size of an organ due to a decrease in the size and number of the cells of which it is composed. Atrophy may be due to physiological or pathological causes. An example of the former is the loss of muscle due to prolonged bed rest, of the latter the wasting of the body in starvation.

See also MUSCULAR ATROPHY, OPTIC ATROPHY.

Autism

A condition beginning in infancy affecting boys rather more commonly than girls, of unknown cause.

The autistic child behaves as if it were alone in the world, growing up and becoming unresponsive to others. Speech is late and is often associated with a frequent repetition of words and phrases. Autistic children may, however, have remarkable memories and have some areas of intellectual activity which are higher than normal even though other areas are grossly retarded.

Babinski's sign

A nervous reflex evoked by a painful stimulus applied to the outer part of the sole of the foot. The stimulus provokes a downward movement of the big toe or plantar flexion, if the nervous system is intact. The presence of this reflex appears to depend particularly on a group of nerve fibres called the pyramidal tracts which pass from the brain to the origin of the motor nerves in the spinal cord, and because these tracts are not fully developed in the human until walking begins, this reflex is not present in a baby.

If the pyramidal tracts are destroyed in an adult at any point along their pathway, for example by cerebral thrombosis, a painful stimulus applied to the outer part of the sole of the foot causes upward movement (dorsiflexion) of the big toe. At the same time the toes spread apart and the flexor muscles of the hip, knee and ankle contract and withdraw the leg from the source of the stimulus. This type of response is often recorded as a positive Babinski sign.

Bacteraemia

The presence of bacteria in the blood stream. These may come from many sources such as boils, dental caries or an infected biliary or urinary system. Commonly the bacteria are only transient and their presence in the blood does not necessarily mean that the normal defence mechanisms of the body have been overwhelmed.

Bacteraemia must be distinguished from the more dangerous condition of SEPTICAEMIA. Nevertheless, bacteraemia may produce clinical effects, e.g. bacteraemia following urethral catheterization may lead to RIGORS, or a bacteraemia occurring in a child who, at the same time, suffers an injury to the growing part of the bone (metaphysis) may result in osteomyelitis.

Bechet's syndrome

An idiopathic form of stomatitis in which chronic aphthous ULCERATION of the mouth and genitalia occur, together with recurrent iritis and ARTHRITIS affecting one or more large joints.

Bell's palsy

A sign of damage to the seventh cranial nerve. In Bell's palsy the whole of the face on the side of the lesion including the forehead is affected, the lower eyelid droops and the angle of the mouth sags. As a result tears flow over the lower lid and an inability to close the eye makes conjunctival damage and infection possible. In addition, because of lack of control of the lips, saliva may dribble from the mouth on the affected side.

The cause of Bell's palsy is unknown. The seventh nerve may, however, be damaged within the cranial cavity by pressure from an acoustic nerve neuroma or in the face below the level of the stylomastoid foramen, by a malignant tumour of the parotid gland.

Bence Jones protein

A protein found in the urine of patients suffering from multiple myelomatosis which is the commonest tumour of bone in man.

This disease is twice as common in men as in women, and usually occurs after the age of 40. It is essentially a cancer of the bone marrow.

The Bence Jones protein is a gamma globulin and its presence in the urine can be demonstrated simply by acidifying the urine and then heating it. Between 60 to 70°C the urine becomes cloudy because the abnormal protein is precipitated, but if the heating is continued it clears as the protein goes back into solution around the boiling point. This simple test is positive in about 50 per cent of patients.

Biliary colic

The pain experienced by a patient suffering from gall stones when a stone is attempting to pass from the gall bladder through the cystic duct into the common bile duct. Like most visceral pains it begins in the epigastrium and then radiates across the upper abdomen and into the back, notably to the angle of the right scapula. The pain is seldom a true COLIC because it is often persistent and of the same severity for several hours. If a stone lodges in the cystic duct it may lead to an acute INFLAMMATION of the gall bladder and should it find its way into the common duct it may obstruct the flow of bile from the liver, causing obstructive JAUNDICE.

Bleeding time

Measurement of the bleeding time measures the response of the small vessels to injury. It is measured in the following way. A small cut is made in the skin of the ear lobe to a depth of 2.5 mm. As soon as the cut is made it begins to bleed and at 30 second intervals the issuing blood is blotted away until the bleeding ceases. The normal time taken for bleeding to cease is between 2 to 5 minutes and the main factors determining this are the contraction of the injured vessels and the clumping together of platelets on the damaged endothelium.

Bleeding time is *not* to be confused with CLOTTING TIME—patients may have a severe clotting defect and a normal bleeding time as in haemophilia.

A prolonged bleeding time is always a sign that the number of platelets in the circulation has been reduced usually below a critical level of about 60 000 per mm^3 as in thrombocytopenic purpura.

Blister

A blister is a collection of serum within the epidermis or in the junction of the epidermis and dermis. The common causes of blisters include:

(1) Friction, e.g. the tight-fitting shoe.
(2) Thermal or chemical injury. The commonest thermal injury is a burn or scald. Severe injuries of this nature may cause the loss of such huge volumes of serum that death occurs from hypovolaemic shock. Chemical blisters often occur in the home due to contamination of the skin with caustic materials.
(3) Infection, e.g. impetigo, pemphigus, chicken pox, herpes zoster and smallpox.

Uncommon causes of blisters include:

(1) Hydroa vaccinoforme, in which blisters occur in response to strong sunlight.
(2) PORPHYRIA, a disease produced by an INBORN ERROR OF METABOLISM.

Blood pressure

The term 'blood pressure' is normally used to describe the arterial blood pressure in a moderately large artery. The blood pressure in other areas is usually prefixed by the name of the vessel in which the pressure is measured, e.g. pulmonary artery pressure, right atrial pressure, etc.

The blood pressure in a large artery has two components, systolic and diastolic. The former is the maximum pressure and is equal to the pressure in the left ventricle immediately prior to the closure of the aortic valves, an event which marks the end of ventricular contraction. Once this has occurred, the onward flow of blood is maintained by the recoil of the elastic tissue in the walls of the larger arteries which has been stretched during the ejection of blood from the heart. As recoil progresses, so the blood pressure gradually falls until it has reached its lowest point, the diastolic pressure, which occurs just prior to the beginning of the next ventricular contraction.

In a normal healthy person the systolic pressure is between 120 to 125 mmHg and the diastolic 75 to 78 mmHg. The gap between the two is the pulse pressure. A gradual increase in pressure occurs with advancing age so that at 70 years of age the systolic pressure may be as high as 170 mmHg and the diastolic 105 mmHg.

At the bedside the blood pressure is normally measured by means of a sphygmomanometer. This consists of an inflatable cuff 13 cm wide which is wound around the upper arm, the bag of which is connected to a mercury manometer. The pressure of air in the cuff is raised by a hand pump, at first to a level exceeding that in the artery. A stethoscope is applied to the artery below the cuff which is then slowly deflated. At first no sound is heard because there is total occlusion of the artery. As the true systolic pressure is reached, an intermittent flow of blood under the cuff commences—intermittent because the flow ceases as the pressure within the artery falls to the diastolic level. This intermittent flow can be recognized by the audible slapping sound which is heard. As the cuff is further deflated the sounds gradually become muffled. This occurs when the pressure in the cuff is equal to the diastolic pressure and when this point has been reached the blood flow through the artery is continuous.

If the blood pressure exceeds normal limits the patient is considered to be HYPERTENSIVE, if below this, HYPOTENSIVE. A patient with a blood pressure within the normal range is often described as normotensive.

Borborygmi

The term used to describe audible bowel sounds. In the majority of individuals these sounds, which are caused by the movement of the intestinal contents, are of little importance, although even in a normal individual excessively audible sounds may occur during stress.

Borborygmi become important, however, if associated with abdominal distension and abdominal COLIC. The sounds then become greatly exaggerated, usually during an attack of pain, indicating the presence of intestinal obstruction.

Absent bowel sounds are also important, indicating the presence of paralytic ileus and the complete cessation of intestinal activity, a condition usually associated with PERITONITIS.

Bradycardia

The heart rate is slower than normal, sometimes as low as 40 beats per minute.

Bradycardia may be:

(1) Physiological: Highly trained athletes, particularly those interested in long distance running may have a heart rate of less than 50 beats per minute.
(2) Pathological.

Pathological causes of bradycardia:

(1) Cardiac conditions:
  (a) Organic disease of the heart causing injury to the conducting system—HEART BLOCK:
    (i) Infective diseases: diphtheria, rheumatic heart disease, scarlet fever and syphilis.
    (ii) Degenerative processes: atherosclerosis of the coronary arteries.
  (b) Drugs: digitalis intoxication.
(2) General conditions:
  (a) Myxoedema.
  (b) JAUNDICE.
  (c) URAEMIA.
(3) INCREASED INTRACRANIAL PRESSURE caused by:
  (a) Tumours of the brain.
  (b) Intracranial HAEMORRHAGE following ruptured aneurysms or trauma.
  (c) Cerebral OEDEMA due to trauma.

Heart block is caused by the interruption of impulses from the atria to the ventricles. If this is complete so that all impulses are blocked, due to the inherent property of cardiac muscle the ventricle continues to contract, but at the rate of about 50 beats per minute, a rate which cannot be increased by exercise.

In myxoedema the cardiac muscle itself is affected and in addition the demand for oxygen and therefore for blood by the body tissues is reduced because of their lowered metabolic rate.

An increase in intracranial pressure causes bradycardia by interfering with the function of the vagus nerves which in part control the normal heart rate.

Bronchial breathing

A sound, heard in the chest, caused by air flowing in and out of the bronchi. In health this sound is damped by the effect of air moving in and out of the alveoli beyond the bronchi. Bronchial breathing is, therefore, normally heard only when this movement of air into the alveoli is abolished, for example by pneumonic consolidation or by blockage of a major bronchus. In the former the alveoli are filled with exudate and inflammatory cells, and in the latter blockage of the bronchus leads to collapse of the lung distal to the obstruction.

Brown-Séquard syndrome

The symptoms and signs which follow the gradual compression of the spinal cord by a spinal tumour. Because the majority of such tumours are asymmetrical in position, the symptoms and signs of the motor disturbance (paralysis) occur on the side of the lesion, whereas loss of sensation to pain, heat and cold occur on the opposite side of the body. This phenomenon occurs because the nerve fibres cross the spinal cord from one side to another almost as soon as they have entered via the posterior spinal roots.

Bruits

The word is derived from a French verb meaning to roar. These are sounds heard over the heart or blood vessels when the circulation becomes turbulent instead of smooth.

Cardiac bruits therefore are usually a sign of valvular disease of the heart. In large arteries, a bruit may be heard when the flow of blood is disturbed by either a narrowing of the vessel by atherosclerosis or external pressure or when dilation has occurred to produce an aneurysm.

Bruits are sometimes heard in diseased tissues in which abnormal quantities of blood are flowing at abnormal speed. An example of this is the bruit heard over the lobes of the thyroid gland in thyrotoxicosis.

Bubo

An enlarged lymph node seen in patients suffering from plague. This disease, the Black Death of the Middle Ages, is caused by a bacterium known as *Pasteurella pestis*. The name is derived from the changes in the infected lymph nodes which may become necrotic and black in colour. *P. pestis* is so virulent that once the infection is established it rapidly invades the blood stream, leading to SEPTICAEMIA and death.

Budd-Chiari syndrome

A syndrome caused by obstruction to the hepatic veins consisting of PORTAL HYPERTENSION, enlargement of the liver and ASCITES. Such obstruction is usually caused by:
  (1) Invasion of the hepatic vein by a hepatic cancer, or metastatic cancer.
  (2) Portal PYAEMIA leading to thrombosis of the hepatic veins.

Cachexia

Extreme wasting of the body tissues, leading to an appearance of extreme emaciation, usually associated with patients dying of advanced cancer.

The causes of cachexia may be obvious. An individual suffering from cancer of the oesophagus starves to death because eventually he suffers from total DYSPHAGIA. A patient suffering from cancer of the stomach also starves to death, either because of complete ANOREXIA or persistent VOMITING due to pyloric stenosis.

Cachexia is commonly associated with severe ANAEMIA which may be due to invasion of the haemopoietic tissues of the bone marrow with metastases or, more commonly, to surface ULCERATION of the tumour followed by chronic blood loss as with carcinoma of the stomach or caecum.

Café au lait spot

Scattered areas of skin hyper-pigmentation due to the local accumulation of melanin in the pigment-forming cells of the dermis known as melanocytes. These scattered pigmented spots are associated with von Recklinghausen's disease in which tumours, known as neurofibroma, develop on the peripheral nerves, spinal nerve roots, nerve plexuses and meninges. Involvement of the nerves supplying the skin results in multiple soft nodules, the skin over which may become pigmented. Von Recklinghausen's disease is usually familial.

Caput medusae

Centrally placed veins forming a cluster around the umbilicus.

The presence of these veins indicates the presence of obstruction to the portal circulation which is usually the result of cirrhosis of the liver.

The veins form part of a collateral circulation allowing the visceral blood, which cannot gain access to the liver and hence to the inferior vena cava, to reach the heart by way of the peripheral veins. The blood flow in a caput medusae is, therefore, from the umbilicus outwards.

Carcinoid syndrome

A rare condition caused by a tumour of the small bowel arising from specialized cells in the mucosa which are able to manufacture a variety of chemical compounds including 5-hydroxytryptamine. These cause excessive DIARRHOEA, BORBORYGMI and intermittent abdominal distension associated with blushing attacks which are often precipitated by alcohol.

Cardiac arrest

The sudden cessation of the heart's action causing a dire emergency because if the circulation of oxygenated blood to the brain is not re-established within 3 to 4 minutes, irreversible changes occur in the vital centres. The patient dies either immediately, or alternatively, survives only by the use of mechanical ventilators.

36

Cardiac arrest may be caused by:

(1) Coronary artery thrombosis causing myocardial infarction and severe cardiogenic shock.
(2) Sudden overactivity of the heart, TACHYCARDIA, caused by emotional excitement or muscular effort in an individual already suffering from myocardial ischaemia.
(3) Severe HAEMORRHAGIC SHOCK.
(4) Disorders in which the serum potassium rises to levels which are toxic to the heart muscle. This is one of the many dangers of severe renal failure.
(5) Over-administration of certain drugs such as adrenaline, quinidine and digitalis.
(6) Electrocution and drowning.
(7) In open-heart surgery the heart is deliberately brought to a standstill but in this procedure the circulation of oxygenated blood to the brain is maintained by artificial means.

Cardiac asthma

A symptom associated with intermittent left ventricular failure in which the affected individual usually wakes at night with a feeling of suffocation whereupon he or she sits up gasping for breath and begins to cough up a pinkish, frothy sputum.

Cardiac asthma only occurs in severe heart failure when the left ventricle fails to contract and empty adequately. In this situation blood is dammed back in the circulation, first in the left atrium and then in the pulmonary circulation. The increased pressure in the pulmonary capillary bed causes the transudation of fluid into the alveoli and so pulmonary OEDEMA.

Oedema of the lungs in turn causes a decrease in the natural elasticity of the lungs so that more muscular work must be done during inspiration, there is a poorer exchange of gases and lastly, because of the fluid entering the bronchial tree, a productive cough develops.

The symptom occurs primarily at night because the adoption of the horizontal position in bed causes an increase in the volume of fluid within the circulation. In a patient with a failing heart this slight increase may be just sufficient to embarrass an already labouring heart.

Cardiac tamponade

A condition in which the action of the heart is endangered by an accumulation of fluid in the pericardial space which lies between the pericardium and the heart itself.

The result of such an accumulation depends upon:

(1) The quantity of fluid.
(2) The speed with which it accumulates. The rapid accumulation of as little as 200 ml may be sufficient to produce symptoms and signs.
(3) The elasticity of the pericardium.
(4) Whether the heart is normal or already diseased.

Cardiac tamponade may be a sign of:

(1) Bacterial or viral pericarditis.
(2) Myocardial infarction.
(3) Stab wounds of the heart.
(4) Open-heart surgery.

The signs of tamponade are an increasing pulse rate, decreasing pulse pressure, muffled heart sounds and an arterial pulse which waxes with expiration and wanes on inspiration, a falling blood pressure followed by death if the condition is not relieved.

These various signs develop because as the pericardial space is filled with fluid so the heart is prevented from filling properly in diastole with the result that the amount of blood ejected from the heart in systole is diminished. Initially the heart is able to compensate for this difficulty by increasing its rate of contraction, hence the rapid pulse, but as the arterial blood pressure falls so the coronary circulation diminishes and with it the blood supply to the myocardium.

Finally the blood flow to the myocardium is insufficient to maintain its normal contractile ability.

Carpo-pedal spasm

A sign of TETANY in which the hands are in a state of painful spasm. The fingers are tightly opposed, flexed at the metacarpo-pharyngeal joints but extended at the interphalangeal, the thumb is flexed and adducted across the palm. Such spasms also occur in the feet but are less obvious, the toes are plantar flexed and the whole foot inverted.

Carpo-pedal spasm develops in any condition in which there is a sudden fall in the plasma concentration of available calcium ion. The low plasma calcium concentration leads to hyper-excitability at the junctions between the motor nerve endings and the muscles.

Among the various causes of carpo-pedal spasm are:

(1) Damage to the parathyroid glands during the operation of thyroidectomy. This reduces the circulating level of parathyroid hormone which controls the level of the circulatory calcium.
(2) Steatorrhoea which results in diminished calcium absorption from the gastrointestinal tract.
(3) ALKALOSIS.

Caseation

A sign of tissue necrosis caused by the bacteria responsible for tuberculosis. Whereas pyogenic bacteria cause a purulent exudate known as pus the tubercle bacillus is associated with the much drier process of caseation.

One of the main features of caseation is the deposition of fatty compounds known as lipids in the tissues which have been destroyed. These are derived from tubercle bacilli themselves.

Caseous material is cheesy in consistency and remains unchanged for long periods unless infected with pyogenic organisms such as the *Staphylococcus aureus*. If infection does not occur, calcium salts are gradually deposited in the caseous material converting the cheesy substance into a hard calcified mass.

Such masses are now rarely seen in the western world in which milk contaminated with the *Mycobacterium* tuberculosis is seldom drunk, but before the heat treatment of milk, caseation and calcified caseous lymph nodes were commonly seen in the cervical region.

Cast or casts

Two of the many meanings of the word 'cast' in the dictionary are to shed or throw off, or to form a certain shape. In medicine, casts are usually moulded to the shape of the organ or part of an organ from which they arise. The most familiar casts are those in the urine which indicate the presence of renal disease.

Casts of renal origin may be composed of:

(1) Cells shed from the renal tubules glued together with urinary proteins (cellular or epithelial casts).
(2) Albumin, erythrocytes and leucocytes (granular casts).
(3) Erythrocytes alone (erythrocyte casts).

Cellular casts are common in the urine of patients suffering from acute nephritis because in this condition the cells of the renal tubules die and are shed into the lumen. When the kidney recovers the casts disappear. If casts continue to appear in the urine it is a sign that the disease has entered a sub-acute or chronic stage. Granular casts are found in any form of renal infection. Erythrocyte casts normally indicate that microscopic haemorrhage is occurring in the kidney.

Catatonia

A sign of severe mental or neurological disturbance in which the sufferer becomes spontaneously immobilized or alternatively remains rigid in a statuesque posture into which he has been placed, however abnormal this may be.

Catatonia is common in schizophrenia, one variant of this illness being known as catatonic schizophrenia. Rarely it is a sign associated with tumours of the frontal lobes of the brain or viral encephalitis lethargica.

Causalgia

A symptom, of unknown aetiology, which may follow an injury to a peripheral nerve in which the chief complaint is one of a severe burning pain in the affected limb. Causalgic pain is often felt beyond the limits of the sensory distribution of damaged nerve, a feature which distinguishes it from the majority of other conditions such as peripheral neuritis which affects the peripheral nerves.

Commonly the skin over the affected part, apart from being extremely sensitive to touch, is red, glossy, hot and even blistered, all signs that the nerves of the autonomic nervous system are involved.

Cerebrospinal otorrhoea

A thin watery discharge from the ear, usually caused by a head injury in which a fracture of the petrous temporal bone has occurred leading to a leak of cerebrospinal fluid to the exterior.

Both cerebrospinal otorrhoea and rhinorrhoea may be complicated by the development of meningitis if infection should make its way through the defect from the exterior. Otorrhoea may also follow infective lesions of the middle ear.

Cerebrospinal rhinorrhoea

A watery discharge flowing from the nose, usually the result of a head injury, causing a fracture of the cribriform plate of the ethmoid together with an associated tear of the underlying dura and arachnoid mater.

Charcot–Marie–Tooth disease

A syndrome in which muscle weakness and wasting appear in the peroneal muscles of the leg, together with loss of sensation. The wasting slowly spreads to involve the anterior tibial muscles and the small muscles of the feet. The severity and distribution of wasting finally lead to the lower limbs assuming the shape of inverted champagne bottles. In the terminal stages the upper limbs are involved and the small muscles of the hand followed by the muscles of the forearm waste. This condition is also known as peroneal muscle ATROPHY and is one of an inherited group of neurological abnormalities.

The underlying cause of the changes remains unknown, although examination of the affected parts of the nervous system shows that various changes have taken place in the anterior horn of the spinal cord and in the ganglia of the sensory nerves.

Cheilosis

The presence of FISSURES and sores around the lips and angles of the mouth. A sign observed in certain vitamin deficiencies such as lack of nicotinic acid or riboflavine.

Cheilosis also develops in healthy individuals exposed to extremely cold dry air and similar lesions occur in herpes, syphilis and lichen planus.

Cheyne–Stokes respiration (periodic respiration)

A repetitive cycle of respiratory activity in 3 phases. First is one of increasingly rapid and deepening breaths, the second is one of slower and shallower movements and the third is a total cessation of respiration (APNOEA), which may last as long as 20 to 30 seconds, after which the cycle is repeated.

This type of respiration can occur in normal neonates and in the elderly, but it is usually regarded as a sign of:

(1) Left-sided HEART FAILURE of sufficient severity to disturb the rhythmical activity of the respiratory centre in the brain stem which controls respiration. This disturbance arises from the alteration in the blood gases which occurs in this condition.

(2) An overdose of sedatives such as barbiturates, which depress the respiratory centre and make it unresponsive to the changes in the blood gas concentrations caused by the poor respiratory movements.

(3) Raised INTRACRANIAL PRESSURE, although the pause in the cycle usually occurs on full inspiration rather than expiration. The increase in intracranial pressure may be caused by:

(a) Intracranial bleeding.
(b) OEDEMA of the brain following head injury.
(c) The growth of a tumour.

As the intracranial pressure rises, so the brain stem (medulla oblongata) and part of the cerebrum are forced through the foramen magnum at the base of the skull, a phenomenon known as coning. This distortion interferes with the blood supply and so causes a disturbance of the vital centres, particularly the respiratory centre. It is this which causes the Cheyne–Stokes respiration.

Chorea

Restless movements of the limbs and body which occur unexpectedly and which may be so severe that the affected person cannot sit or stand. Choreiform movements are non-repetitive and may merely be gross exaggerations of intended movements, characteristics which distinguish them from a TIC.

The presence of chorea is a sign of an organic lesion of the brain, but there is no agreement as to which particular part must be damaged in order to produce such abnormal movements.

Chorea occurs in:

(1) Acute rheumatism caused by the haemolytic streptococcus.
(2) In children suffering from brain damage due to:
    (a) Birth injury.
    (b) Oxygen deprivation.
    (c) KERNICTERUS.
(3) In adults suffering from organic brain damage due to cerebral atherosclerosis or brain tumours.
(4) Huntington's chorea which occurs in the fourth and fifth decades, and in addition to the involuntary movements is associated with progressive DEMENTIA.

Chvostek's sign

Hyper-excitability of the facial muscles in patients suffering from TETANY demonstrated by tapping the facial nerve as it emerges from the base of the skull just below the mastoid process.

Claudication

A severe cramp-like pain, most commonly felt in the muscles of the buttocks or calves, brought on by exercise which is a sign of a diminished supply of blood to the affected limb. Once claudication begins it becomes worse if the exercise is continued, until finally the patient is forced to a halt and from that moment the pain begins to diminish in intensity. The distance the patient can walk prior to the onset of pain gives some idea of the flow deficiency.

The common causes of a decreased flow of blood to the lower limb and therefore of claudication include:

(1) Atherosclerosis of the aorta, iliac or femoral arteries.

(2) Thrombo-angiitis obliterans, Buerger's disease.
(3) Injury to an artery sufficiently severe to reduce the blood supply to the limb.

The cause of the pain is unknown but it is generally believed to be due to a metabolite produced by exercise which is not removed from the muscle mass when the circulation is poor. This chemical compound, structure unknown, has become known as the P factor. The cessation of exercise allows the residual circulation to clear this factor from the muscles.

The limb of the patient often shows other evidence of a diminished blood flow including wasting, lack of hairs, dryness of the skin, CYANOSIS and sometimes ULCERATION or GANGRENE.

A similar pain may occur in the lower limb after exercise when the deep venous circulation has been damaged. Unlike claudication, however, this pain is described by the patient as bursting in character and is not relieved by ceasing to exercise the limb unless it is also raised thereby assisting venous drainage.

Clay-coloured faeces

A sign that bile pigments have not passed from the bile duct into the gastrointestinal tract. Hence clay-coloured stools will be present in any patient suffering from JAUNDICE in whom the cause is obstructive regardless of the point of obstruction. The gradual return of normal colour to the stools usually indicates relief of the obstruction.

Clonus

The abnormal response of a muscle to stretching, in which a series of rhythmic contractions occur instead of a single contraction.

Clonus is a sign that the cortico-spinal (pyramidal) nerve tracts which descend from the motor cortex of the brain to the anterior horn cells of the spinal cord have been damaged at some point in their pathway either within the brain or spinal cord. Such damage is usually due to:
(1) Injury.
(2) Insufficient blood supply to some part of the brain or

spinal cord which is usually the result of thrombosis of the arterial supply to these areas.

(3) The presence of tumours compressing the tracts.

Clonus in the quadriceps muscle of the thigh can be detected by placing the patient on his back and then quickly pushing the patella towards the foot. This movement stretches the quadriceps muscle and will cause rhythmical contractions to occur if there is damage to the appropriate part of the cortico-spinal tract.

Since clonus is a sign of a pyramidal tract disorder it is always accompanied by grossly exaggerated tendon reflexes in the affected part. In the example quoted, it would be anticipated that the knee jerk would be abnormal.

Clotting and clotting time

Clotting describes the process whereby blood changes from its normal fluid consistency to a more solid jelly-like substance known as a clot. Clotting normally occurs within blood vessels if the flow becomes stagnant or when blood escapes from the vascular system into the tissues. Blood removed from the circulation also clots and the rapidity with which this occurs measures the clotting time.

Clotting is a complex chemical process involving a large number of chemical substances known as the clotting factors and, in addition, the presence of an adequate number of platelets, vitamin K and calcium. If any of these are absent or deficient, clotting cannot occur and the result is a group of diseases collectively known as the clotting disorders. The classical examples are HAEMOPHILIA, which is due to a deficiency of clotting Factor VIII, and Christmas disease due to a deficiency of Factor IX. Both these conditions are congenital hereditary disorders. In addition, acquired deficiencies of the clotting mechanisms may develop including hypofibrinogenaemia due to severe liver disease or extensive intravascular clotting. The latter is an occasional complication of severe injuries or certain obstetrical complications such as abruptio placentae.

The normal time taken for blood to clot when removed from the body varies between 5 to 11 minutes.

45

Coffee-ground vomiting

A specific sign of bleeding from the stomach or duodenum. Coffee-ground VOMITING only occurs when the blood has been retained in the stomach long enough for it to be partially digested by the gastric juice.

The common causes of upper intestinal bleeding include:

(1) Chronic duodenal ULCERATION.
(2) Acute gastric erosions.
(3) Chronic gastric ulceration.
(4) Oesophageal varices.
(5) A miscellaneous group of causes including hiatus hernia and cancer of the stomach.

When the bleeding is so rapid that the blood is vomited prior to digestion the term HAEMATEMESIS is used. In either situation SHOCK may develop if more than 0.5 to 1 litre of blood has been lost.

Colic

A type of pain caused by the violent, intermittent contraction of the smooth muscle surrounding certain abdominal organs such as the ureter, the bile duct, small and large intestine. The presence of colic usually indicates that the lumen of the affected organ has become obstructed.

The distribution of colicky pain makes the source relatively easy to identify, e.g.:

(1) Renal colic begins in the loin and passes down to the pubis.
(2) Small bowel colic is usually centred around the umbilicus.
(3) Large bowel colic is below the level of the umbilicus.
(4) Appendicular colic begins around the umbilicus.

If, in addition to obstruction, the affected organ also becomes inflamed, the intensity of the colicky pain usually increases. This occurs because INFLAMMATION increases the sensitivity of the nerve endings in the affected organ which thus respond with greater intensity to the stimulus of distension.

A good example of this is the condition of acute appendicitis in which the initial or central abdominal pain gradually increases in severity as the lumen of the organ is first obstructed and later inflamed.

See also BILIARY COLIC, GALL BLADDER COLIC, URETERIC COLIC.

Coma

A state of prolonged unconsciousness, gradual in onset, from which spontaneous recovery does not occur, coma is usually a sign associated with:

(1) Diseases affecting the brain or its coverings such as cerebral thrombosis, encephalitis or a severe head injury.
(2) Metabolic disorders affecting cerebral function such as URAEMIA, diabetes mellitus and hepatic failure.
(3) Acute barbiturate, alcohol and salicylate poisoning.
(4) Miscellaneous conditions including heat exhaustion.

In coma the patient does not react to verbal or painful stimuli; the tendon, plantar, corneal and pupillary reflexes are depressed or absent and CHEYNE–STOKES type of respiration is common.

Concussion

A sign accompanying moderate or severe head injury in which a state of unconsciousness occurs, the duration and depth of which are related to the severity of the injury.

Concussion is caused by the 'shaking' of the brain, like a jelly, within the bony cranium. This motion probably causes spasm or even tearing of the small blood vessels supplying the nerve cells of the brain.

Concussion is always associated with some loss of memory (AMNESIA) both for events which precede the injury (retrograde amnesia) and events following the injury (post-traumatic amnesia). In the majority of patients both are usually of short duration but, following severe damage and a prolonged period of concussion, the amnesia may last for weeks or months.

Constipation

The retention of faecal matter within the colon and rectum so that the bowels are open less often than normally, a situation which leads to the passage of dry, hard stools known as scybala. Constipation may be caused by:

(1) Delay in the passage of faecal matter along the colon due to diminished intestinal peristalsis. This is natural in old age but it also occurs in healthy individuals if the bulk of the faeces is reduced by:

   (a) An inappropriate diet which contains too little roughage.
   (b) The excessive removal of water from the faeces. This is a common cause of constipation in tropical climates or in patients suffering from a fever with its attendant sweating and DEHYDRATION.

Delay in faecal transit may also be the result of:

   (a) Endocrine causes such as myxoedema and panhypopituitarism.
   (b) Incomplete innervation of the colon, Hirschsprung's disease.
   (c) Idiopathic megacolon, see ABDOMINAL SWELLING.
   (d) Anatomical obstruction of the colon. A cancer of the colon eventually causes obstruction to the passage of faeces but this type of constipation is normally associated with abdominal COLIC, BORBORYGMI and ABDOMINAL SWELLING.

The passage of neither flatus nor faeces is often referred to as absolute constipation.

(2) Delay in emptying the rectum. Defaecation is stimulated by the intermittent entry of faeces into the rectum. This normally occurs after eating through the action of the gastrocolic reflex which is initiated by the post-prandial stretching of the stomach wall. The faecal mass distends the rectum, stimulates the nerve endings in its wall and gives rise to the urge to defaecate. If such impulses are ignored the sensation of fullness dies away even though the faeces remain. The gradual absorption of water from the faecal mass leads to a harder stool which becomes increasingly difficult to evacuate. Spurious DIARRHOEA may follow.

(3) When defaecation is painful due to the presence of such

conditions as a FISSURE in ano or painful haemorrhoids the natural desire to defaecate is suppressed.

Contusion

A sign of an injury caused by a blunt object striking the body with sufficient force to rupture the small subcutaneous blood vessels without breaking the skin surface. This type of injury causes bruising because the red blood cells leak into the inter-stitial tissues from the damaged blood vessels and liberate their pigment, haemoglobin.

The term contusion can be applied even to an injury, the result of which is invisible so long as only minimal vascular damage has occurred, e.g. a contusion of the brain tissue fol-lowing a head injury.

Convulsion see FIT

The terms convulsion and fit are interchangeable and are used to describe attacks of involuntary movements of the limbs, trunk and face which may or may not be associated with loss of consciousness.

Cor pulmonale

A term used to describe the various symptoms and signs associ-ated with right-sided HEART FAILURE which is usually the end result of severe pulmonary disorders such as chronic bronchi-tis, emphysema and asthma.

Each of these conditions leads to changes in the lung tissues which result in diminished elasticity and difficulty in transfer-ring the oxygen and carbon dioxide from the air in the lungs to the blood and vice versa. In addition changes occur in the small blood vessels of the lung causing increasing resistance to the flow of blood through the lungs which also contributes to the inadequate oxygenation of the blood.

As a result of this increasing resistance in the pulmonary circulation the right ventricle is eventually unable to drive blood through the lungs in sufficient quantity to prevent the development of CYANOSIS.

The symptoms of cor pulmonale include increasing DYSP-NOEA and COUGH, the latter usually being worse in winter when exacerbations of the underlying pulmonary disease occur. As the condition deteriorates increasing cyanosis and respiratory difficulty develop. Because movements of the chest wall are limited by the underlying disease, the accessory muscles of respiration in the neck are used to assist inspiration, the patient is now a 'blue bloater' usually OBESE, cyanosed and unhappy.

Cough

A violent expulsion of air from the lungs. A cough may be a symptom associated with many diverse conditions including:

(1) Diseases of the respiratory tract, commonly of an inflammatory nature.
(2) HYSTERIA.
(3) Irritation of the recurrent laryngeal nerves.
(4) HEART FAILURE.
(5) Infection of the paranasal air sinuses.
(6) Accidental inhalation of fluid or a foreign body into the respiratory tract.

A cough consists of 3 actions which must follow one another in a co-ordinated manner:

(1) A deep inspiration followed by closure of the larynx.
(2) A rise in the intrathoracic pressure produced by a contraction of the chest and abdominal muscles.
(3) An abrupt release of this pressure by a sudden opening of the closed glottis.

If as a result of coughing sputum is produced the cough is termed productive. The underlying cause of a cough can frequently be discerned by first listening to the cough and then examining the sputum. Thus in tracheitis the cough is frequent but dry, the 'hacking' cough. In acute bronchitis the cough is severe and the sputum mucopurulent, purulent or mucoid depending upon the stage of the disease. In lobar pneumonia the sputum is sparse but 'rusty' in colour because of the altered blood which it contains and in heart failure the cough is often nocturnal, frothy and blood stained. A cough which results in the production of large quantities of foul fetid sputum suggests the presence of bronchiectasis, a lung ABSCESS or severe tuberculosis with superimposed secondary infection.

Cramp

Cramp is a lay term used to describe painful and excessive contractions of the skeletal muscles. The affected muscle group is extremely painful, feels hard and 'knotted' and even when relaxation occurs considerable residual tenderness remains.

Studies of this condition have shown that the excessive muscular contraction which provokes the sensation of a cramp is due to the motor units which initiate contraction by firing impulses in a completely disorganized manner.

Cramps are a symptom of many clinical conditions including:

(1) Excessive fatigue in normal muscles, presumably due to the retention of metabolites which are not washed out of the muscle by the blood.

(2) Cramps, especially in bed at night, occur in elderly people with no obvious physical disease.

(3) Following excessive sweating, the result of exposure, occupation or disease. Presumably due to decreased salt content disorganizing the electrical activity at the nerve end plates in the muscle.

(4) When the serum calcium is low, causing TETANY.

(5) In tetanus due to the liberation of tetanus exotoxin by the *B. tetani*.

(6) Due to some poisons, e.g. strychnine.

(7) Due to decreased blood supply to the muscles, causing intermittent CLAUDICATION.

Crepitus

A sign present in a number of different conditions indicating:

(1) Disease of joints. Movement of any joint in which the articular cartilage has been destroyed is accompanied by crepitus, a grating sensation caused by the diseased articular surfaces rubbing against one another.

(2) A fracture. A similar grating sensation will be felt when a fracture line is disturbed. This sign is rarely deliberately elicited since it would not only cause severe pain, but also it might increase the actual or potential displacement of the fracture line.

51

(3) The presence of gas in the tissues. This imparts a crackling sensation to the palpating fingers. The common causes of gas in the tissues are:

(a) Injuries of the chest leading to a communication between the lung tissue or the air passages themselves, and the subcutaneous tissues of the chest wall. Such a communication may follow a stab wound or fracture of a rib. The subcutaneous tissues become infiltrated with air, a condition known as surgical emphysema.

(b) Perforation of a hollow viscus which communicates with the subcutaneous tissues. An example of this is the development of surgical emphysema of the neck following accidental perforation of the oesophagus.

(c) Infection of the subcutaneous tissues with gas-forming organisms. This condition known as gas GANGRENE, is caused by infection of damaged tissues with the anaerobic clostridial bacteria. This infection is rare because these bacteria multiply only in a completely oxygen-free environment. Gas gangrene, therefore, only develops in wounds in which large masses of soft tissue have been destroyed, blood vessels have been damaged and the wound is heavily contaminated with faeces. Two varieties of clostridia are involved; the first, of which *Cl. welchii* is an example, produces exotoxins which actually kill the tissues, and the second, an example of which is *Cl. hystolyticum*, causes putrefaction and breaks down the tissue proteins into foul-smelling products the chief of which are the gases hydrogen, hydrogen sulphide and carbon dioxide. During the process of putrefaction the affected muscles change from brick-red to greenish-black in colour.

(4) The presence of OEDEMA of the lungs or INFLAMMATION of lung tissue. In either of these conditions by the use of a stethoscope or an ear applied to the chest it is possible to hear sounds to which the name crepitation is

applied. This sound can be imitated by rubbing a lock of hair between the forefinger and thumb in close proximity to the external auditory meatus. The sound is produced by air entering the fluid-filled terminal air spaces and it is most clearly heard when the patient breathes deeply towards the end of inspiration.

The commonest cause of pulmonary oedema is congestive HEART FAILURE, and the common cause of inflammation is either a viral or bacterial pneumonia.

Crigler–Najjar syndrome

A rare inherited disorder usually manifesting itself in the newborn in which the enzyme responsible for certain changes in the bile pigment bilirubin is absent. As a result bilirubin leaks into the brain tissue and causes severe brain damage (KERNICTERUS).

In milder degrees both changed and unchanged bilirubin may be present in the plasma and in these babies serious brain damage may not necessarily occur.

Crisis

Strictly interpreted the term crisis means the sign of a turning point for better or worse in the course of an illness although it is now used in a variety of ways:

(1) In its original sense prior to the introduction of antibiotics, patients suffering from lobar pneumonia would often undergo a remarkable and sudden change, the crisis, usually 5 to 10 days from the onset of the disease. The patient, hitherto CYANOSED, DYSPNOEIC, febrile and DELIRIOUS would suddenly improve within a matter of hours and the temperature would fall to a more normal level.

(2) Metabolic states which may become rapidly worse within a few hours:

(a) The thyroid crisis or storm. Common in the past but now rare, a thyroid crisis occurs in patients subjected to the operation of thyroidectomy who have been improperly prepared for surgery. The affected individual suddenly develops FEVER, TACHYCARDIA, agitation and finally CARDIAC FAILURE, usually within 48 hours of operation. The cause remains uncertain but is probably due to an excess of circulating thyroid hormone liberated during the operation.

(b) Adrenal crisis. An adrenal crisis is precipitated by a sudden decrease in the circulating level of adrenocortical hormones. This may be the result of:

  (i) Destruction of the adrenals by natural disease—the WATERHOUSE–FRIDERICHSEN SYNDROME.
  (ii) Removal of the adrenals, adrenalectomy, without adequate replacement therapy.
  (iii) Intercurrent infection in a patient in whom an adrenalectomy has been performed but who is thrown out of balance as a result of the infection.
  (iv) Sudden withdrawal of steroids in a patient who has undergone prolonged treatment with these drugs.

The clinical features of an adrenal crisis are the rapid onset of NAUSEA, VOMITING, abdominal and muscular pains and profound hypotension. If this condition is unrecognized, death is inevitable, but when proper replacement therapy is given, survival is probable.

(c) Diabetic crisis. The sudden onset of severe ketoacidosis in a diabetic patient. The common causes include a dry tongue, intense thirst and polyuria, con- by the inadequate administration of insulin or its substitutes or the development of intercurrent infection. Glucose metabolism becomes upset and as a result, KETOSIS develops. The clinical symptoms include, a dry tongue, intense thirst and polyuria, constipation, muscle CRAMPS and altered vision, although there may be no alteration in consciousness. Hypotension and long deep sighing 'acidotic' respiration develop. Acetone can be smelt on the breath and ketone bodies are found in the urine. The blood sugar is usually extremely high. A diabetic crisis is treated by rehydration with intravenous fluids, the correction of the metabolic ACIDOSIS and the promotion of normal glucose metabolism by the administration of adequate doses of insulin.

(3) Visceral crisis:
   (a) Dietl's crisis. Attacks of severe renal pain, possibly produced by movements of the kidney. These obstruct the pelvi-ureteric junction and so temporarily prevent the outflow of urine from the kidney.
   (b) Gastric crises of tabes. The sudden attacks of severe upper abdominal pain occasionally occur in patients suffering from late syphilis. These attacks are similar to the commoner 'lightning' pains in the upper thighs. The mechanism of the pain is unknown.

Crush syndrome

A particular form of injury in which considerable masses of muscle tissue have been damaged.

The main signs associated with this syndrome which distinguish it from a simple injury are:

(1) The injured person remains remarkably well until the crushing agent is removed, after which SHOCK rapidly develops followed by renal failure.
(2) Once the crushing agent is removed the injured limb becomes swollen, tense and weak.

The underlying cause of shock in this syndrome is the increase in capillary permeability which occurs in the damaged muscles, thus allowing large quantities of protein-rich fluid to escape into the tissues. The blood volume is thus reduced causing hypovolaemia.

In addition the muscle pigment, myoglobin, is liberated into the circulation and this increases the amount of renal damage which is already taking place because of the renal ischaemia caused by the hypovolaemic shock.

Cushingoid appearance

The descriptive term applied to the appearance of an individual in whom excessive amounts of adrenocortical hormones are circulating in the body.

An excess of this group of hormones causes certain effects the chief of which are:

(1) A large round face, often referred to as a 'moon' face.
(2) Excessive deposition of fat, particularly on the trunk and proximal parts of the limbs.
(3) HYPERTENSION, an abnormally high blood pressure.
(4) Osteoporosis which is a state in which there is a deficiency of bone without alteration of its quality or architectural arrangement; this change causes increasing KYPHOSIS.
(5) In the female, AMENORRHOEA, hoarseness of the voice and HIRSUTISM.

The commonest cause of a cushingoid appearance is the over-administration of steriod hormones in the treatment of diseases such as rheumatoid arthritis.

Less common are:

(1) The presence of a basophil tumour of the anterior hypophysis (pituitary) which stimulates the adrenals to produce excessive quantities of steroids (Cushing's disease).
(2) Hyperplasia or a tumour of the adrenal cortex itself, causing Cushing's syndrome. If this tumour is malignant the cushingoid woman is nearly always VIRILIZED.

Cushing's syndrome see CUSHINGOID APPEARANCE

Cyanosis

A blue or bluish coloration of the skin, mucous membranes or deeper organs usually observed in the face, hands, feet, mucosae or deep structures.

Cyanosis is a sign of severe oxygen deficiency, but to be present at all a minimum concentration of 5 g of reduced (de-oxygenated) haemoglobin must be present in the circulation. Should a patient be so anaemic that the total content of haemoglobin is below this level, cyanosis would not be observed.

56

A common classification of the causes of cyanosis is:

(1) Peripheral: If the rate of blood flow through the capillaries is reduced, more time is available for the removal of oxygen from haemoglobin by the tissues. This state of affairs may result from:
   (a) Local causes, exposure to cold.
   (b) Factors reducing the cardiac output, such as SHOCK or HEART FAILURE.

(2) Central: In this type of cyanosis there is an excess amount of reduced haemoglobin in the blood leaving the heart. This might arise in the following manner:
   (a) The lungs may be so affected by disease that the blood flowing through them cannot be oxygenated. This may result from pneumonia or chronic bronchitis when large areas of the lungs may be inadequately ventilated even though blood continues to flow through them.
   (b) The ventilatory capacity, i.e. the amount of movement of the chest wall may be so reduced that the overall efficiency of the lungs is impaired as in poliomyelitis.
   (c) Blood may be shunted from the right side of the heart to the left without passing through the lungs. This is the cause of cyanosis in septal defects in the heart such as Fallot's tetralogy in which the following cardiac abnormalities are present:
      (i) There is a defect in the base of the interventricular septum and the aorta arises from both ventricles above this defect.
      (ii) The pulmonary valve is stenosed (smaller than normal).
      (iii) The right ventricle is hypertrophied.

(3) Polycythaemia, an increase in the number of circulating red cells, may be accompanied by cyanosis due to the incapacity of the lungs to oxygenate all the excess haemoglobin content of the blood.

In addition to true cyanosis due to the presence of normal but reduced haemoglobin in the blood, an apparent cyanosis may occur if abnormal pigments are present in the circulation such as sulphahaemoglobin or methaemoglobin, neither of which can carry oxygen. Reduction of haemoglobin to methaemoglobin is usually the result of the ingestion of drugs such as sulphonamides or analgesic drugs.

Deafness

Loss of hearing which is of two types:

(1) Conductive deafness caused by blockage of the external meatus or disease of the middle ear. In this group any sound except for the patient's own voice is heard with difficulty although there is no distortion and if the sound is amplified it may become audible.

(2) Perceptive or sensori-neural deafness resulting from a defect in the inner ear or in the nerve pathways leading from the inner ear to the brain. In this type of deafness the hearing loss tends to affect varying frequencies. Since the individual cannot hear his own voice speech normally deteriorates, e.g. the patient may appear to shout unnecessarily. Individuals suffering from perceptive deafness usually have difficulty in hearing a conversation carried out against a background noise.

These two forms of deafness can be distinguished by the simple tuning fork test, Weber's test and audiometry.

In Weber's test, the base of a vibrating tuning fork is applied to the top of the head in the midline. In a normal individual the sound is transmitted equally to the inner ear on both sides of the skull. When an individual suffers perceptive deafness the vibration is heard better in the ear with the better function but in conductive deafness, the sound is transmitted to the ear with the greater conductive loss.

Common causes of conductive deafness include wax in the external auditory meatus, foreign bodies or otitis media with or without perforation of the drum.

Causes of perceptive deafness include Ménière's disease, acoustic nerve neuroma, excessive exposure to abnormal noise levels, the effect of certain drugs such as streptomycin and infections involving the eighth nerve such as pyogenic meningitis.

The commonest cause of congenital acquired deafness is infection of the mother with rubella (German measles) especially during the first 3 months of pregnancy.

Defaecation

The passage of faeces or stools from the body. Faeces consist of 70 to 80 per cent water, bacteria, mucus, epithelial cells, undigested and indigestible food residues derived from vegetables and cereals, salts derived from the intestinal secretions and bile pigments of various kinds.

The rectum is normally empty but faeces are pushed at intervals by the action of the colonic muscles into the rectum. This usually occurs after a meal through the action of the gastro-colic reflex, food distending the stomach exciting a reflex which causes the colon to contract.

As the faecal mass distends the rectum and stimulates sensory nerve endings, impulses pass to the central nervous system in a normal person and give rise to an urge to defaecate. At this point the anal sphincter muscles relax and faeces are forced out of the body by the peristaltic movement of the pelvic colon. This action may be assisted by contracting the diaphragm and muscles of the abdominal wall, thus increasing the intra-abdominal pressure and so exerting increasing force upon the faecal mass.

In the baby defaecation is a reflex action and it returns to a reflex action in a person who is unconscious or who cannot consciously control the requisite reflexes because of spinal cord injury.

In old age where rectal sensation may be reduced, the faecal mass fails to wake any sensation of fullness, with the result that it remains in the rectum, giving rise to spurious DIAR-RHOEA.

Defibrination syndrome

A dangerous haemorrhagic state caused by excessive CLOTTING within the blood stream. The available plasma fibrinogen is used up faster than it can be replaced with the result that the blood in the circulation cannot clot and so unexpected bleeding occurs.

This rare syndrome is occasionally seen in the mother following premature separation of the placenta, after the administration of a mis-matched blood transfusion, in the course of overwhelming infection, in malignant disease and following cardiac or prostatic operations. A similar condition is also produced by the bite of the Malayan pit viper, the venom of which contains an enzyme which destroys fibrinogens.

Dehydration

A sign indicating a reduction in the water and salt content of the body usually presenting with a 'drawn' face, dry tongue and wrinkled skin, but as the condition progresses the patient develops hypovolaemic SHOCK.

The common causes of dehydration include:

(1) Excessive VOMITING from any cause.
(2) Excessive gastric aspiration.
(3) Loss of fluid and salt from intestinal FISTULA.
(4) Severe DIARRHOEA.
(5) Prolonged pyrexia.
(6) Evaporation of body fluid from a severe burn.
(7) Inadequate intake of fluid, due to DYSPHAGIA.

Milder degrees of dehydration may be corrected by the oral administration of salt and water, but if severe, intravenous therapy is required.

Occasionally dehydration is deliberately induced, as in the treatment of cerebral OEDEMA resulting from a head injury where there is swelling of the brain and INCREASING INTRACRANIAL PRESSURE. If this situation is allowed to progress, death may occur and so diuretic drugs are administered in order to cause shrinkage of the brain tissue and hence a reduction in the intracranial pressure.

Delirium

A state of partial unconsciousness which is accompanied by restlessness of both the body and mind. Such a state may be associated with the severe cerebral lesions which may accompany injuries to the brain due either to trauma or vascular accidents, or it may be caused by acute fevers of infective origin even though the brain itself is not involved. Thus, typhoid fever, septicaemia and rickettsial infections are commonly accompanied by delirium, as is FEVER from any cause in elderly patients.

Delusion

A symptom of mental disorder, occurring with great frequency in patients suffering from schizophrenia.

A delusion is a belief which is not true to fact, cannot be corrected by logical argument and is out of keeping with a patient's education and surroundings. The common delusions relate to ideas of grandeur, persecution or disease.

Dementia

A symptom indicating a generalized decay of mental function in which intellect, memory, thought, emotion and behaviour are all affected.

An early sign may be an abnormal response to a given situation, a response usually representing an unexpected error of judgement. Later memory is impaired and uncharacteristic mood patterns occur followed finally by APHASIA, APRAXIA and agnosis. The most frequent cause of dementia is atrophy of brain tissue caused by atherosclerosis of the cerebral blood vessels. Less common causes include syphilis, alcoholism and metabolic disorders such as myxoedema.

Diarrhoea

A symptom implying the too frequent passage of fluid or semi-solid faeces from the bowel. The opposite of CONSTIPATION.

Precisely what constitutes diarrhoea varies in different ethnic groups, in the West defaecation seldom occurs more than once a day whereas in the Bantu living in a rural society a diet of mealies will predispose to 6 or 7 stools a day because of the high fibre content. Furthermore, in the same ethnic group defaecation differs at the extremes of age, a normal baby commonly defaecates after each feed but does not suffer from diarrhoea.

The causes of diarrhoea are many but the commonest are:
(1) Dietary factors—food stuffs containing too much fibre may cause diarrhoea.

(2) Infection. Infection of the 'food poisoning' type by *Salmonella* or specific infections such as typhoid, cholera, bacillary dysentery.
(3) Diseases of the pancreas or small bowel giving rise to incomplete fat digestion and, therefore, bulky stools, STEATORRHOEA.
(4) Inflammatory conditions of the large bowel, e.g. ulcerative colitis, amoebic dysentery.
(5) Excess intake of magnesium salts—a patient suffering from a duodenal ulcer may unwittingly self-administer too large a dose of magnesium salts (iatrogenic diarrhoea).
(6) Cancer of the large bowel which is often associated with intermittent constipation and diarrhoea. Large papilliferous tumours may secrete great quantities of mucus and this leads to the frequent passage of stools containing little but mucus.
(7) Antibiotics which may destroy the normal bacteriological flora of the bowel and superimposed infections occur leading to diarrhoea (post-antibiotic diarrhoea).

Rarer causes of diarrhoea include endocrine disorders such as thyrotoxicosis.

It is also possible for the severely constipated patient to suffer diarrhoea but in this case the condition is referred to as 'spurious'. It is due to retention of increasing amounts of hard faeces in the rectum which stimulates the mucous membrane to secrete excessive quantities of mucus which are then passed through the anal sphincter as a dirty brown faecal discharge. This condition is relatively common in old age and may sometimes occur following illnesses which have led to DEHYDRATION.

Diplopia

The seeing of 2 instead of one visual image, which can only occur if the brain receives 2 separate visual images.

Rarely double vision arises because of an abnormality within the eye itself; for example a traumatic dislocation of the lens may result in some light rays passing through the lens and others to the side so that 2 images fall on the retina. More commonly, however, double vision is a symptom of squint (strabismus) although a squint is not necessarily associated with diplopia.

A paralytic squint is associated with impaired movement of the eye or eyes and, if not immediately obvious becomes so on attempting to turn the eye in the direction of the paralysed muscle. When, for example, the function of the sixth cranial nerve, which innervates the external rectus muscle of the eye, is deranged or the muscle itself is damaged by disease diplopia occurs only on looking sideways, because this muscle is concerned with external rotation of the eye. The subsequent images are seen by the affected individual to lie in a horizontal plane, in other words side by side. The sudden development of a paralytic squint in the absence of a history of injury may be the result of a wide variety of diseases involving especially the cardiovascular, central nervous and endocrine systems, all of which may affect the nerves controlling ocular movements or even the muscles themselves.

A concomitant or non-paralytic squint occurs in individuals in whom the external muscles of the eye are working but in whom there is a breakdown in the cerebral mechanisms which fuse the images normally presented to the brain. This ability to fuse the visual images usually develops within the first 6 months of life. If it is not acquired the child learns to suppress one unwanted image and when this is continued over a period of weeks or months the disuse of the visual mechanism finally leads to a deterioration of visual acuity, AMBLYOPIA, which may become permanent.

Discharge, vaginal see VAGINAL DISCHARGE

Dislocation

A term most frequently applied to a joint indicating that the articulating surfaces of the joint have completely separated so that one is no longer in contact with the other. Dislocations occur when the tissues which normally hold the articular surfaces together such as the capsule, ligaments and surrounding muscles, are damaged or deficient.

Dislocation may be:
(1) Congenital, e.g. congenital dislocation of the hip.
(2) Acquired:
  (a) Traumatic. The jaw and shoulder joints are commonly dislocated by injury. Occasionally a traumatic disturbance may cause severe damage to the blood vessels and/or nerves in the region of the joint. A joint such as the shoulder once dislocated, frequently dislocates with increasing ease on future occasions even though the force applied may be less. This is due to the shallowness of the joint. This can be compared with dislocations of the hip joint which are frequently complicated by fractures of the acetabulum.
  (b) Dislocation is sometimes a sign of some underlying pathological process. For example, destruction of the joint by an acute INFLAMMATORY process such as a septic arthritis frequently leads to dislocation.

Disorientation

A disorder of consciousness in which the individual no longer appreciates his relationship with other individuals or with time or place.

Disorientation of topographical type in which the individual is unable to recall a clear mental picture of a familiar route or the internal layout of a familiar building is often a symptom associated with tumours or ATROPHY of the parietal lobe of the brain. Involvement of the right parietal lobe by similar conditions may lead to imperception of the left half of the body so that its position and movement are unrecognized. Elderly patients are commonly disoriented after surgery due to a combination of cerebral atrophy, sedation and cerebral ANOXIA.

Distension

A term which is usually applied to the distended abdomen observed in patients suffering from intestinal obstruction. However, any hollow or tubular organ may become obstructed with the result that the viscus or tube proximal to the obstruction becomes distended. Thus, the veins around the umbilicus, when distended form the CAPUT MEDUSAE, signifying obstruction to the portal system of veins. Distension of the jugular veins of the neck may indicate mechanical obstruction to the return of blood to the heart due to the presence of an intrathoracic tumour, or there may be obstruction to the return of blood to the heart due to CARDIAC FAILURE.

Diuresis

The production of increased quantities of urine which is a common sign of:

(1) Psychological disturbance. Any severe emotional disturbance may be followed by a diuresis which is due to a decreased secretion of antidiuretic hormone (ADH) by the posterior lobe of the pituitary gland.

(2) Physiological disturbance. When a normal individual drinks a volume of fluid in excess of his needs a diuresis follows. This is because cells known as chemoreceptors in the carotid body which is situated at the bifurcation of the common carotid artery, sense that the blood is becoming diluted as the excessive fluid is absorbed. This information is passed to the brain with the result that the secretion of the antidiuretic hormone (ADH) is reduced.

(3) Pathological disturbance:

    (a) Destruction of the posterior part of the pituitary gland or interference with the base of the brain near the stalk of this gland by tumours, vascular accidents or surgical interference may lead to a complete lack of the antidiuretic hormone (ADH). This is followed by the condition known as diabetes insipidus in which as much as 20 litres of urine a day may form. Such a diuresis is accompanied by severe polyuria and thirst.

    (b) Renal conditions. Diuresis is always associated with diseases of the kidney which are accompanied by damage to the renal tubules because in the presence of tubular damage, the reabsorption of water into the blood stream is impossible.

(c) Diabetes mellitus. In this disease excessive quantities of sugar filter through the glomeruli into the tubules and this retains the water in the tubules causing the condition known as an osmotic diuresis.

A diuresis also accompanies the use of certain drugs such as frusemide which acts on the tubule cells to prevent the re-absorption of water. Known as the diuretics these compounds are particularly valuable in the treatment of patients suffering from HEART FAILURE who have developed OEDEMA.

Down's syndrome

The most common autosomal disorder in which most of the infants possess 47 instead of 46 chromosomes in each cell, the affected chromosome being number 21 hence the alternative name of trisomy 21.

In mothers of 25 years of age, Down's syndrome occurs once in every 2000 live births, but the risk increases 40-fold by the age of 45 years.

The diagnosis is made by the appearance of the child. The head is often small with a flat occiput, high cheek bones and small flattened nose, the eyes are slanted upwards laterally, the tongue is large and tends to protrude from the small mouth, the hands are short and broad and possess only one transverse palmar crease and congenital heart disease and atresia of the duodenum are common.

Varying degrees of mental handicap become evident as the infant grows, the I.Q. being usually below 50.

Dubin–Johnson syndrome

An inherited condition presenting usually in early adult life with attacks of JAUNDICE, associated with dark urine and upper abdominal pain. The stools may be pale and the liver may be enlarged or tender. The underlying cause of the syndrome is an inability of the liver cells to secrete bilirubin which is, there-fore, regurgitated from the liver cells back into the plasma.

Dysarthria

A disturbance of speech due to an inability to articulate. Dysarthria occurs when the function of the lips, tongue or palate either separately or together is disturbed. Characteristically the disturbance of speech affects the enunciation of the consonants and not the vowels.

It may be due to local disease or mechanical defects of these structures as in the individual suffering from a cleft palate. Perhaps the commonest temporary cause of dysarthria is a visit to the dentist which is accompanied by a local anaesthetic affecting the lips and the tongue, an inferior dental block. Until the effects of the anaesthetic pass off the affected individual has great difficulty in articulating.

Dysarthria may also be the result of neurological disorders such as poliomyelitis or motor neurone disease affecting the various nuclei from which the cranial nerves supplying the lips, tongue or palate arise. Tumours at the base of the brain affecting the 12th (hypoglossal) nerve which supplies the tongue are particularly associated with difficulty in enunciating the 'r' sound. Seventh (facial) nerve palsies are particularly associated with difficulties in the pronunciation of 'p', 'b' and 'm'. Myasthenia gravis, which is also associated with PTOSIS, may cause marked dysarthria which becomes worse with the passage of time.

Articulation also suffers in diseases such as Parkinson's disease or conditions affecting the cerebellum.

Dyschezia

Rectal insensibility of such severe degree that defaecation is not initiated by a full rectum.

The call to defaecate in a normal individual originates in a sensation of rectal fullness but this can only arise when the rectum is sensitive to distension. In the elderly rectal sensation is reduced and so DIARRHOEA due to leakage of mucus past the faecal mass occurs. Rarely dyschezia is due to an organic lesion such as a fracture of the spine, which by causing damage to the spinal cord or cauda equina cuts off rectal sensation.

Dyslexia

A symptom of a functional disorder of the brain, the precise cause of which remains unknown.

The major problem is difficulty in reading occurring in a child of average or above average intelligence. Unrecognized dyslexia may persist into adult life. The condition is often associated with mirror writing in which words are written down as if they were being viewed in a mirror.

Dysmenorrhoea

Painful menstruation. Usually divided into two types:

(1) Pain of uterine origin occurring at the time of menstruation; this type is known as true, primary, spasmodic or intrinsic and arises usually on the first day of the period. It is due to uterine contractions and is therefore colicky in nature and felt mainly in the hypogastrium and possibly the thighs.

True dysmenorrhoea is often divided into primary and secondary varieties according to whether it begins with the menarche (the commencement of menstruation) or later in life. The cause of true dysmenorrhoea occuring early in the reproductive period of life is a matter for speculation, but it is probably due to hormonal imbalance, particularly related to the excretion of progesterone, since if the uterus is not exposed to the influence of this hormone, as in anovular bleeding, pain does not occur. True dysmenorrhoea may also be caused by organic conditions, these include:

  (a) the passage of large clots during menstruation, rarely seen except in association with MENORRHAGIA.
  (b) The presence of an intrauterine contraceptive device.
  (c) The presence of submucous uterine myomata.

(2) Congestive dysmenorrhoea. This type usually is associated with pain during the two or three days which precede menstruation and it is usually slowly relieved after its onset. It is often associated with menorrhagia and is commonly accompanied by backache. The cause may be increasing tension in the pelvic tissues due to premenstrual engorgement. In the majority of patients no organic abnormality can be demonstrated, but in some patients there may be chronic infection of the ovaries and tubes.

In women over the age of 30 dysmenorrhoea may arise due to the disease of endometriosis. In this condition the pain varies in position according to the site of the disease and usually begins with premenstrual aching for 2 or 3 days, reaching its climax during or at the end of the period when the abnormally placed endometrium is menstruating into itself. Unlike true spasmodic dysmenorrhoea the pain persists throughout the period and ceases only when menstruation ends.

Dysphagia

Difficulty in swallowing which is a symptom of many diseases:
  (1) Conditions involving the oropharyngeal region.

    (a) Painful conditions such as tonsillitis, Vincent's angina and diphtheria may make swallowing temporarily difficult.
    (b) Affections of the cranial nerves which innervate the muscles concerned in swallowing.
        (i) Bulbar palsy: A condition arising from degeneration of the nerve cells giving origin to the last 4 cranial nerves. The initial symptom is usually dysarthria and only later in the disease does dysphagia develop.
        (ii) Poliomyelitis.
        (iii) Myasthenia gravis in which the actual abnormality causing the dysphagia lies at the junction of the motor nerve with the muscle, i.e. at the motor end plate.

(2) Conditions affecting the oesophagus itself. When oesophageal obstruction is present the act of swallowing may be normal but the food is felt to stick at some point between the sternal notch and the lower end of the sternum. The causes may be congenital or acquired.

   (a) Congenital: Atresia of the oesophagus, a rare condition seen in the neonate in which feeding is accompanied by regurgitation and respiratory difficulty.

   (b) Acquired: *Causes involving the wall of the oesophagus:*

      (i) Carcinoma of the oesophagus.
      (ii) Strictures of the oesophagus caused either by the swallowing of corrosives or the action of acid gastric juice. The latter occurs in the presence of a hiatus hernia in which the oesophago-gastric junction is incompetent, it is usually preceded by a long history of HEARTBURN.
      (iii) Pharyngeal diverticulum, the development of which is usually associated with a long history of malfunction of the sphincter lying at the upper end of the oesophagus.
      (iv) Pharyngeal webs associated with the Plummer–Vinson syndrome.
      (v) Achalasia of the cardia in which the lower end of the oesophagus fails to relax.

   (c) Acquired: *Causes producing extrinsic pressure on the oesophagus:*

      (i) Malignant metastatic mediastinal lymph nodes.
      (ii) Pressure from a dilated atherosclerotic aorta, dysphagia lusoria.
      (iii) An enlarged heart as in left ventricular HEART FAILURE.

In many patients suffering from oesophageal dysphagia the cause and the site can be accurately predicted from the clinical history. Organic obstruction usually causes a slowly developing dysphagia because well-chewed solid food can still be swaling dysphagia because well-chewed solid food can still be swallowed even when the lumen of the gullet has been reduced to 5 mm in diameter. The dysphagia is, therefore, usually first noted when swallowing solids and only later when swallowing liquids. Long-standing dysphagia is associated with CACHEXIA.

Dyspnoea

An undue awareness of respiratory effort, often described by the patient as fighting for breath.

Normal individuals subjected to excessive or violent exercise do develop dyspnoea although the severity of the exercise required to produce breathlessness varies according to the degree of physical fitness. Exercise increases the tissue demand for oxygen, which is provided by increasing the cardiac output and both the rate and depth of respiration.

Dyspnoea is a prominent symptom of:

(1) Cardiac disorders particularly those associated with failing function of the left ventricle such as occurs in mitral stenosis. Factors contributing to the onset of dyspnoea in cardiac conditions include:

(a) Pulmonary congestion and OEDEMA which cause the lungs to become increasingly turgid so that inspiration requires a greater physical effort. As this effort increases so the accessory muscles of respiration come into action. The degree of congestion is related to posture. Increasing pulmonary congestion occurs in the horizontal position due to a movement of blood from the splanchnic circulation in the abdomen to the pulmonary circulation in the thorax. This is the main reason why individuals suffering from CARDIAC FAILURE sleep in the sitting position and wake if they slip down the bed. When such congestion is complicated by bronchospasm the degree of dyspnoea worsens producing the condition known as CARDIAC ASTHMA.

(b) Stimulation of the collection of nerve cells in the brain stem which form the respiratory centre. These cells are sensitive to the falling oxygen content of the blood and the rising concentration of carbon dioxide. An increasing rate of discharge from this centre increases both the rate and depth of respiration.

(2) Pulmonary disorders. Chronic pulmonary conditions such as emphysema and chronic bronchitis when sufficiently advanced lead to a slowly progressive dyspnoea due to increasing difficulty of gaseous exchange in the diseased lung tissue. Similarly space-occupying lesions in the chest such as a pneumothorax, pleural effusion or mediastinal tumour may lead to dyspnoea due to interference with cardiac activity and an actual reduction in the amount of lung tissue available for gaseous exchange.

(3) Anaemia. Severe anaemia from any cause will eventually precipitate dyspnoea due to the decreasing ability of the blood to carry oxygen. Unlike the cardio-respiratory cripple who prefers to sit up or lie propped up the dyspnoeic anaemic patient often prefers to lie flat.

Dysuria

Painful frequent micturition.

The commonest cause of dysuria is a Gram-negative bacterial infection of the lower urinary tract which includes the bladder and urethra in the female or the bladder, prostate and urethra in the male. Other less common causes of dysuria include infection by tuberculosis and *Bilharzia haematobium*, the latter being particularly common in Africa, Egypt and Iraq.

Dysuria is more frequent in females than in males because the female urethra is short and, therefore, ascending infection is commoner and in addition the female urethra may be injured during sexual intercourse. In the majority of sexually active women infection is limited to the complex glands surrounding the urethra, hence the term the 'urethral syndrome'. In such women the mid-stream specimen of urine is usually sterile. In males in whom dysuria is less common it is frequently secondary to incomplete emptying of the bladder which may be caused either by benign or malignant prostatic enlargement, or less commonly by a urethral stricture.

In either sex the bladder becomes infected in the presence

of a malignant bladder tumour and also occasionally dysuria is caused by infection from adjacent infected viscera lying in close proximity to the bladder such as the colon or Fallopian tubes.

Earache

Denotes pain in the ear which may be due to:

    (1) An INFLAMMATION involving the external ear which is the commonest cause and can be produced by:

        (a) Injury.
        (b) Impetigo.
        (c) Gout.
        (d) Meatal boils.
        (e) Foreign body.
        (f) Tumours in the region of the meatus.

        Any inflammatory lesion involving the meatal tissues such as a boil or insect bite produces extremely severe pain because the tension in the involved tissues becomes rapidly excessive due to their density.

    (2) Conditions involving the middle ear, mainly otitis media and acute mastoiditis, the latter now being extremely rare due to the introduction of antibiotics.

    (3) REFERRED PAIN in the ear may arise from a variety of sources because the nerve supply to the ear is extensive, being derived from the 5th, 9th, and 10th cranial nerves as well as from the 2nd and 3rd cervical nerves.

        Common causes of referred pain therefore include unerupted molar teeth, cancer of the tonsil or naso-pharynx and glandular enlargement in the neck.

    (4) Pain due to actual involvement of nerves is caused by tic douloureux, herpes zoster and, very rarely, syphilis, associated with the condition of tabes dorsalis.

Ecchymosis

Diffuse flat HAEMORRHAGES into the skin, mucous membranes or viscera.

    The presence of an ecchymosis is usually a sign of injury. Rarely they are caused by a bleeding disorder caused either by a platelet defect as in primary thrombocytopenic purpura or by weakness of the capillary wall. An example of the latter is the disease of scurvy in which a lack of vitamin C causes disintegration of the capillary walls.

Eisenmenger's syndrome

A condition in which increasing pressure in the pulmonary circulation leads to blood passing from the right side of the heart to the left in patients in whom, because of septal defect and patent ductus arteriosus, the normal flow of blood would have been from the left side of the heart to the right side. Such patients usually have no symptoms during childhood, but in adolescence or early adult life CYANOSIS and FINGER CLUBBING develop. The prognosis is poor and death may occur suddenly or following HEART FAILURE.

Encephalopathy, hepatic see HEPATIC ENCEPHALOPATHY

Enophthalmos

Recession of the eye into the body orbit, a change which may be unilateral or bilateral depending on the cause.

The commonest cause of unilateral enophthalmos is displacement of the bones of the orbit as a result of injury. Less commonly enophthalmos is due to paralysis of the muscles at the back of the orbit, the loss of tone allowing the eye to recede. These muscles are supplied by the sympathetic nervous system and this may be interrupted in a variety of ways.

(1) By malignant tumours in the neck such as cancers of the thyroid gland or metastatic disease in the cervical lymph nodes. Either may invade and destroy the sympathetic trunk.

(2) By injury to the nerves of the brachial plexus by which route the sympathetic nerve fibres emerge from the spinal cord.

(3) By surgical injury. Deliberate excision of part of the sympathetic nerve chain is required in some patients suffering from Raynaud's phenomenon or excessive sweating of the hand (HYPERHYDROSIS). This operation is known as cervical sympathectomy.

Sympathetic damage causing enophthalmos is frequently associated with narrowing of the palpebral FISSURE due to drooping of the upper eyelid (PTOSIS) and constriction of the pupil on the affected side (meiosis).

Eosinophilia

A sign normally associated with allergic disorders such as asthma, skin conditions such as pemphigus and parasitic infections such as hydatid disease.

Eosinophilia itself is not associated with symptoms and it is discovered only on routine examination of the blood film in patients suffering from the diseases such as those already mentioned or related conditions. In a normal individual the eosinophilic white cells represent only between 1 and 6 per cent of the total white cell count. In eosinophilia the count greatly exceeds this.

Epigastric pain

Pain in the epigastric or subcostal region is a symptom commonly associated with diseases of the viscera occupying the upper abdomen. However, it must never be forgotten that acute, as opposed to chronic or recurring, epigastric discomfort may occur following such diverse conditions as a myocardial infarction, herpes zoster (shingles) or diaphragmatic pleurisy.

The common causes of chronic intermittent abdominal pain include such conditions as:

(1) FUNCTIONAL dyspepsia. A condition in which all investigations designed to prove the presence of organic disease are negative. This type of epigastric pain is often poorly localized, vague in character, bears little relationship to meals and is often accompanied by bizarre symptoms.

(2) Duodenal ULCERATION. The pain associated with this condition is usually well localized and associated with tenderness to the right of the midline. The pain is frequently provoked by hunger and relieved by food and drink. The factors responsible for this pain are exposure of the ulcerated surface to acid and the accompanying spasm of the smooth muscle at the pyloric end of the stomach.

75

(3) Hiatus hernia. Although sometimes associated with epigastric pain, this condition most commonly presents with HEARTBURN. The pain is often provoked by stooping, the wearing of tight garments or pregnancy, all of which raise the intra-abdominal pressure.

(4) Gall stones. The pain associated with gall stones is seldom colicky despite frequent references in the literature to BILIARY COLIC. Precipitated perhaps by fatty meals, the pain is usually poorly localized. Acute INFLAMMATION of the gall bladder is associated with more definite upper ABDOMINAL PAIN, together with FEVER.

Epistaxis

Whilst the commonest cause of nose bleeding is injury or infection it may also be a prominent sign of general disorders such as:

(1) Blood diseases:
   (a) Conditions leading to a critical shortage of platelets and thus a prolonged BLEEDING TIME such as primary or secondary thrombocytopenia.
   (b) Conditions associated with coagulation defects such as HAEMOPHILIA or Christmas disease, or a prolonged prothrombin time such as occurs in obstructive JAUNDICE.

(2) Vascular disorders:
   (a) Hereditary telangiectasia, a hereditary vascular defect associated with the presence of multiple vascular naevi formed by grossly dilated capillaries.
   (b) Von Willebrand's disease, a hereditary disorder characterized by a prolonged bleeding time, low plasma concentration of Factor VIII and failure of the capillaries to contract when injured.
   (c) Defects in the capillary wall such as occur in vitamin C deficiency (scurvy), bleeding from the gums is somewhat more common than epistaxis in this condition.
   (d) Bacterial and viral infections which may be associ-

ated with nose bleeding because of damage to the capillary walls.

Epistaxis is also relatively common in hypertensive patients although it is difficult to demonstrate any anatomical changes in the small blood vessels of the nose.

Erythema

A reddening of the skin caused by dilatation of the arterioles and capillaries. In normal individuals the local flushing of the face is an erythema based upon an emotional response. Pathological erythema is a sign of FEVER, superficial burning or acute INFLAMMATION in all of which vasodilatation occurs.

Erythromelagia

A term used to describe red, painful extremities which are also hot and sweat excessively.

The majority of cases are idiopathic but occasionally erythromelagia is a sign of HYPERTENSION, or disease of the peripheral nerves due to metallic poisoning, nutritional deficiency and arterial disease.

Euphoria

An abnormal feeling of physical and mental well-being for which there is no reason. A symptom occurring in many conditions although how it is caused is uncertain.

Euphoria is a prominent symptom in about a quarter of patients suffering from multiple sclerosis. It also occurs in patients suffering from lesions of the frontal lobes of the brain caused by HAEMORRHAGE, tumour or surgery. It may also occur in patients suffering from incurable malignant disease even though no actual organic lesion can be demonstrated in the brain.

Exophthalmos

Protrusion of the eye from the orbit to a greater degree than normal, the reverse of ENOPHTHALMOS.

The condition may be unilateral or bilateral according to the underlying cause and in rare cases the presence of abnormal blood vessels lying behind the eye leads to a condition known as pulsating exophthalmos due to the pulsation being transmitted to the eye.

The commonest cause of bilateral exophthalmos is overactivity of the thyroid, thyrotoxicosis, in which the protrusion is caused by OEDEMA and infiltration of the orbital fat by lymphocytes. Similar changes occurring in the external occular muscles may lead to weakness and so a diminution in the range of movement of the eyes (external exophthalmic ophthalmoplegia), a condition associated with DIPLOPIA. Advanced exophthalmos may leave the cornea of the eye totally unprotected. When the eyelids cannot be closed, corneal ULCERATION and blindness may then follow.

Unilateral exophthalmos is usually caused by orbital or retro-orbital tumours. The rare pulsating exophthalmos is always due to injuries of the head which have been complicated by the development of a communication between the cavernous sinus and the internal carotid artery which lie behind the orbit.

Extrasystoles

An alteration in the heart beat associated with organic heart disease, usually of ischaemic origin due to atherosclerosis. The symptoms are PALPITATION, or an awareness of a missed heart beat.

Extrasystoles arise when a heart beat is initiated by a focus other than in the sino-atrial node. The abnormal area of origin may be in the wall of the atrium, the atrio-ventricular node or even the ventricles themselves.

The contraction of the myocardium initiated by the abnormal stimulus usually occurs at a fixed time interval following the preceding normally stimulated heart beat and causes only a feeble contraction. Nevertheless after the 'ectopic' beat a long pause follows because the myocardium cannot be stimulated again for some time. It is because of this that the affected individual may be aware of a missed beat. Palpation of the radial artery at this time reveals an abnormally prolonged interval between two pulses.

Extravasation

The escape of blood from the vascular system into the tissues resulting in an ECCHYMOSIS, bruise or HAEMATOMA according to the severity of the bleeding. Injury leading to extravasation may be made worse by:

(1) A platelet deficiency such as occurs in primary or secondary thrombocytopenia which causes an increase in the BLEEDING TIME.

(2) A total or relative absence of clotting factors from the blood such as occurs in HAEMOPHILIA.

An extravasation of urine may also occur, usually from the bladder or prostatic urethra and nearly always due to deliberate or accidental trauma. Thus a fracture of the pelvis leading to rupture of the urethra at the junction of the prostatic and membranous parts may be followed by a leakage of urine into the pelvic connective tissue planes. If nothing is done to relieve the situation a suprapubic swelling gradually develops.

Fainting

A transient loss of consciousness often preceded by giddiness, NAUSEA and a feeling of extreme weakness. This is the lay term for syncope.

A faint is caused by a temporary diminution in the supply of blood to the brain and vital centres caused by a fall in the cardiac output. The causes of a sudden fall in cardiac output, and therefore of fainting, include:

(1) The vaso-vagal attack. These attacks usually occur when an individual is subjected to pain or a powerful emotion such as fear. The vagus nerve is stimulated via the higher centres, the heart rate is suddenly reduced and cardiac output falls, and because the vital centres are rendered temporarily anoxic, the patient faints. These attacks nearly always occur in the standing position and, therefore, if unpleasant information which may frighten or horrify a patient or relative has to be imparted, be sure they are sitting down first.

(2) Primary cardiac disease. An abrupt reduction in cardiac output may follow a myocardial infarct (heart attack)

particularly if the heart should stop beating altogether or pass into a state of ventricular fibrillation. Similarly in patients suffering from cardiac disease, a sudden change in rhythm, as for example when a normally beating heart passes into heart block, may diminish the cardiac output. These attacks are often known as STOKES–ADAMS ATTACKS.

(3) Excessive straining on defaecation or micturition can raise the intrathoracic pressure to such a level that venous return to the heart is impeded.

(4) Pooling of blood in the peripheral circulation. This is the cause of postural fainting such as occurs in the soldier standing to attention for too long a period on the parade ground. Blood pools in the vessels in the lower half of the body, the venous return falls and so eventually the soldier faints. Having fallen to the ground in the horizontal position the blood is redistributed and recovery occurs.

(5) The excessive administration of some antihypertensive drugs or vasodilators.

A faint must be distinguished from:

(1) The fit of epilepsy.
(2) HYSTERIA.
(3) HYPOGLYCAEMIA.
(4) The 'drop' attacks which occur in association with atherosclerosis of the cerebral blood vessels which are precipitated by spasm in the diseased arteries.

Fever

A term indicating the presence of a rise in the body temperature above the accepted normal of 37°C.

The causes may be divided into:

(1) Infective—when the infecting agent is either by bacteria or viruses.

(2) Non-infective. A wide variety of different diseases may be associated with pyrexia including:

    (a) Malignancy, almost any malignant tumour may be associated with a fever. The fever associated with

Hodgkin's lymphoma is often very characteristic and is associated with cycles of relapse and remission each of which last from 7 to 10 days. This is known as the Pel-Ebstein fever.

(b) 'Immunological' disorders associated with fever include acute rheumatic fever, rheumatoid ARTHRITIS, progressive systemic sclerosis.

(c) Severe anaemia, a haemoglobin level below g/dl may be associated with fever.

(d) Endocrine disorders, particularly thyrotoxicosis. In the thyroid crisis which may follow infection in an untreated thyrotoxic patient or surgery in an improperly prepared patient the temperature may rise to 39°C.

(3) Unknown origin, P.U.O. A pyrexia of unknown origin still occasionally occurs when even after death no apparent cause can be found to account for the fever present during life.

Fever due to infection is due to the production by the infecting agent of chemical substances known as pyrogens, or fever-producing substances. In addition once infection has become established endogenous pyrogens are produced from the damaged tissue cells, notably the polymorphonuclear leucocytes which maintain or enhance the temperature level attained. Both types of fever-producing substance produce their effect by acting on the heat-regulating centre at the base of the brain.

Fevers are often described as continuous when the daily fluctuations in temperature are less than 1°C, remittent when the daily fluctuation is more than 1°C but a normal temperature is never reached, and lastly intermittent when the temperature swings by more than 1°C but falls to normal at some point in the day.

Finger clubbing—hypertrophic pulmonary arthropathy

A particular appearance of the fingers in which the terminal portions of the fingers and/or toes swell so that eventually the affected digits resemble drum sticks. The nail also increases in

81

convexity in both directions and commonly the affected digits are warmer than normal.

This deformity typically occurs in patients suffering from certain forms of chronic pulmonary disease which include:

(1) Cancer of the lung, mediastinum or pleura. Ten per cent of patients suffering from cancer of the bronchus develop clubbed fingers.

(2) Chronic infections of the respiratory system such as bronchiectasis.

These various changes in the fingers are caused by OEDEMA of the subcutaneous tissues, thickening of the digital blood vessels and proliferation of the connective tissue cells which itself leads to an increased deposition of collagen; only in severe cases do changes also occur in the bones.

Why these various pathological changes occur is uncertain. It has been suggested that they result from toxins formed by the underlying primary lesion or by obscure autonomic nerve REFLEXES causing vasodilation of the digital blood vessels. In addition, finger clubbing may be inherited in otherwise normal individuals and it may very rarely be an isolated finding in the absence of any family history.

Fissure

A break, usually narrow like a crevice, in the continuity of an epithelial surface.

Examples of common fissures are:

(1) Anal fissures which develop in the anal canal due to tearing of the epithelial lining by the passage of an excessively hard stool. This type of fissure is exceedingly painful and produces severe spasm of the sphincter muscles of the anus. Increasing fear of the painful defaecation makes the patient increasingly CONSTIPATED.

(2) CHEILOSIS—fissures around the lips. The common predisposing causes include viral infections and vitamin deficiencies, a less common cause is syphilis.

Fistula

A fistula is an abnormal communication between 2 hollow viscera or between a hollow viscus and the surface. All relatively new fistulae are lined by granulation tissues but long-standing communications may eventually develop an epithelial lining.

Examples of fistulae:

(1) Between hollow viscera:

    (a) Gastro-colic fistula—A communication between the stomach and colon which is usually caused by a cancer of either viscus which has invaded its neighbour or by chronic ULCERATION of the stomach involving the colon. The usual symptoms associated with such fistulae are severe DIARRHOEA caused by faecal contamination of the upper gastrointestinal tract and CACHEXIA due to malabsorption.

    (b) Vesico-colic fistula—A communication between the sigmoid colon and bladder. The commonest cause is diverticulitis, and, less common is cancer of the colon. Symptoms include recurrent frequency and pain on micturition (DYSURIA) caused by infection and the passage of flatus per urethram.

    (c) Entero-colic fistula—A communication between the small bowel and colon. The common causes are chronic inflammatory conditions of the wall of the bowel (Crohn's disease) or cancer. Common symptoms include severe DIARRHOEA and weight loss due to malabsorption.

(2) Between a hollow viscus and the surface:

    (a) Fistula-in-ano—A communication between the anal canal and the peri-anal skin. Common causes include a previous FISSURE in ano or peri-anal or ischiorectal ABSCESS. Symptoms include severe peri-anal discharge and itching.

    (b) Faecal fistula—A communication between the small bowel or colon and the surface of the abdominal wall. These are commonly caused by inflammatory and neoplastic diseases of the bowel or by break-down of a surgical anastomosis. Common symptoms include leakage of intestinal contents on to the abdominal wall. This may be followed by

DEHYDRATION and excoriation of the abdominal wall skin.

Fit

A fit is the popular name for a CONVULSION or sudden violent involuntary muscle contraction, however caused.

Fits may be:

(1) Idiopathic, the cause is unknown as in idiopathic epilepsy.
(2) Symptomatic, a demonstrable cause may be present in some part of the brain such as an intracranial tumour, cerebral atherosclerosis, the scar of a previous injury to the brain or infections such as meningitis or encephalitis.
(3) Hysterical, fits precipitated by an emotional crisis never occur during sleep and the patient is never hurt. The attack is often prolonged in front of an interested audience.
(4) Metabolic, fits are not uncommon in HYPOGLYCAEMIA, URAEMIA and hepatic failure.
(5) Due to toxins. Fits may follow poisoning with matrazol, some insecticides and lead.
(6) Withdrawal fits. The withdrawal of any drug such as alcohol or barbiturates to which a patient has become habituated may be followed by fits.

Flaccid paralysis

A form of paralysis of striated skeletal muscle caused by injury to the motor nerves supplying the affected muscles at any point from their origin in the spinal cord to their junction with the muscle itself at the motor end plate.

In this type of paralysis the muscles are flabby, flaccid and undergo severe wasting. The tendon reflexes are either diminished or absent.

The causes of a flaccid paralysis include:

(1) Poliomyelitis. In areas of the world in which poliomyelitis (a viral infection) is common and the poliomyelitis vaccine is not available this disease will be the commonest cause of flaccid paralysis.

84

(2) Spinal injury. Although a spinal injury does not produce a permanent flaccid paralysis of the muscles below the level of the spinal cord lesion the immediate effect is to do so, this stage is known as the stage of spinal SHOCK and lasts for between one to 3 weeks. Similarly, IN-FLAMMATION of the spinal cord may cause a flaccid paralysis, such inflammation may be due to viruses, multiple sclerosis or syphilis.

(3) Progressive muscular ATROPHY, a rare disorder usually affecting men over 40 years of age in which degeneration of the nerve cells in the spinal cord occurs together with degeneration of the corresponding nerve fibres.

(4) Injury to specific nerves, e.g. an injury to the ulnar nerve which supplies the majority of the muscles of the hand leads to gross wasting of the small muscles of the hand and corresponding loss of function.

(5) Peripheral neuropathy. This condition which usually affects more than one nerve may be a manifestation of numerous infections (bacterial or viral), metabolic disorders such as diabetes, dietary deficiencies such as beriberi and metallic poisoning especially with compounds of lead, arsenic and mercury. However, in this condition the effects of the disease usually begin in the distal parts of the limb and slowly spread proximally. Commonly motor and sensory fibres are affected equally so that in addition to the flaccid paralysis there is also loss of sensation.

Flatulence

Gaseous distension of the upper gastrointestinal tract often associated with excessive eructation (belching). Unrelieved flatulence causes an intense bloated feeling in the upper abdomen. Fortunately most individuals can belch with relative ease and this is particularly so in patients suffering from a hiatus hernia in whom the mechanisms preventing the reflux of gastric contents into the oesophagus have been destroyed.

Flatulence is common in normal individuals after dietary or alcoholic indiscretion and in individuals suffering from peptic ulceration, gall stones or ANXIETY or neurosis.

Focal epilepsy

A form of epilepsy consisting of a localized FIT usually without any loss of consciousness.

The convulsive movements usually commence in the same group of muscles on each occasion and then gradually extend usually in a proximal direction, frequently involving one limb but occasionally extending to involve the whole of one side of the body or even to produce a generalized CONVULSION. This type of epilepsy is a sign of a focal disturbance in the cerebral cortex and the severity of the attack is only limited by the spread of the disturbance across the brain.

Occasional attacks of similar nature are secondary to various conditions which cause cerebral damage including:

(1) Birth injuries.
(2) Closed head injuries associated with depressed fractures of the skull.
(3) Infective conditions such as syphilis or encephalitis.
(4) Atherosclerosis of cerebral vessels causing a cerebral infarct or degeneration.

Folie à deux

A symptom associated with paranoid schizophrenia in which the sufferers impose their own DELUSIONS on normal persons who accept them as being founded on reality. This situation usually only arises in persons living in close proximity with one another.

Formication

A rare symptom in which the patient describes a sensation as if worms or insects were crawling under the skin.

Patients suffering from TETANY due to hypocalcaemia or over-breathing sometimes describe this type of sensation. The exact cause is unknown.

Fortification spectra

Bright jagged streaks of light usually seen by a patient at the beginning of a migrainous attack which may last from 10 to 20 minutes, to be later followed by the typical migrainous HEADACHE.

86

The mechanism of such visual displays is uncertain although it may be the result of vascular changes at some point along the visual pathways.

Frequency of micturition

Pedantically this section should be entitled 'increased' frequency of micturition. This symptom has many causes and it is important to know how much urine the patient passes on each occasion.

(1) Polyuria. If increasing amounts of urine are being formed by the kidneys an increased frequency of micturition will occur because the bladder is filled more rapidly and, therefore, the desire to micturate will occur more frequently than normal. The diagnosis becomes obvious when it is realized that the patient is passing abnormal quantities of urine, approximately 250 to 300 ml on each occasion. Polyuria occurs following an increased intake of fluid, or in certain pathological conditions, notably diabetes mellitus, diabetes insipidus or chronic renal disease.

(2) More commonly an increased frequency of micturition involves the passing of smaller than normal quantities of urine at very frequent intervals. The causes of true frequency include:

(a) ANXIETY.

(b) INFLAMMATION or irritation of the bladder or urethra, or both. An inflamed irritated bladder responds by contraction to minimal degrees of distension, so causing the desire to empty the bladder at frequent intervals. Inflammation of the bladder is usually associated with pain, the combination of painful frequency often being referred to as STRANGURY. Inflammation of the bladder is usually caused by bacteria, usually of the coliform group.

Cystitis may be primary, there being no other pathological condition present, or secondary to obstruction to the normal passage of urine. The latter may be caused by prostatic enlargement, stones in the bladder or tumours around the bladder neck.

'Cystitis' in the absence of any underlying cause is common in sexually active women in whom the condition is often referred to as the urethral syndrome.

Other causes of frequency include:

(3) Enlargement of the prostate gland in males leading to an inability to empty the bladder completely. This may cause frequency even in the absence of infection.

(4) Irritation of the bladder by a vesical calculus. In the absence of infection, this type of frequency is often less severe in bed at night because the stone rolls away from the sensitive base of the bladder.

(5) Pressure on the bladder by growths of the surrounding organs. The enlarging uterus in early pregnancy may produce frequency of micturition, as also may pressure on the bladder by massive fibroids of the uterus.

(6) Diminution in the size of the bladder. This is usually the result of chronic infection which may cause fibrosis and therefore shrinkage of the bladder wall. This group includes tuberculosis, now rare in Western society, Hunner's ulcer, a rare condition always found in women and bilharzia, a parasitic infection common in the East.

Frohlich's syndrome

A rare disorder in children, in which OBESITY and lack of genital development occur, caused by tumours in the region of the hypothalamus which interfere with the function of the hypophysis. The hypothalamic lesion is the underlying cause of the obesity whilst the hypogonadism is due to a deficiency of the hormone group known as the gonadotrophins.

Frostbite

A vascular lesion following exposure to extreme cold which usually affects the extremities or the face. There is damage to the lining of the arterioles and venules (the endothelium) with the result that thrombosis of the blood inside the vessel occurs. In severe cases, ice crystals may actually form in the cells of the surrounding tissues. As the part becomes frozen sensation diminishes, the affected part becomes brittle and at first is usually pale, although sometime later it may become blue due to the reduction of the oxyhaemoglobin in the stagnant capillaries.

When the affected individual is removed to a warm environment those blood vessels not completely destroyed dilate and the skin becomes hot, red and painful. Fluid escapes from the affected vessels (transudation) and the affected part becomes swollen with OEDEMA and blistered. This stage is usually completed in one to 2 weeks after which the affected part returns to normal. If actual thrombosis occurs, total recovery is impossible and GANGRENE of the affected part occurs.

Fugue

A symptom associated with HYSTERIA. A hysterical individual may leave home, behave in an apparently rational manner but recovery has complete AMNESIA for the whole episode.

Functional

When the symptoms and signs of which a patient complains result from a disorder of the mind the condition is classified as functional. For example, a singer facing her first engagement in front of a critical audience may develop a hysterical APHONIA, losing her voice without any organic disease of the larynx being present.

Gait, alterations in

Watching the manner in which an individual walks, his gait, often assists an observer to discern the cause of a patient's disability. The gait may be disturbed by a soft tissue or bony lesion situated anywhere from the undersurface of the foot to the level of the lumbar spine. It may also be affected by injury or disease of the central or peripheral nervous system involving either the motor or sensory pathways.

Typical abnormalities of the gait caused by disease of the nervous system include:

(1) The HIGH-STEPPING GAIT following foot-drop, the common causes of which are prolapse of an intervertebral disc and peripheral neuropathy. A similar type of gait

is caused by loss of position sense (proprioception) in the lower limbs as occurs in syphilitic infection of the central nervous system causing tabes dorsalis, or in the neuropathy associated with vitamin B_{12} deficiency in which sub-acute combined degeneration of the cord occurs.

(2) A staggering gait. Such a gait is caused by lesions involving either the cerebellum or vestibular apparatus. The affected individual is unsteady and walks with the feet wider apart than a normal individual. When the causative lesion affects only one side the patient staggers towards the affected side when trying to walk in a straight line.

(3) A shuffling gait which is common in PARKINSONISM. It is frequently an early sign of this disease which is caused by degeneration of various parts of the brain. Characteristic of this type of gait is an absence of associated arm movements when walking.

(4) A spastic gait. A type seen following a STROKE complicated by HEMIPLEGIA. Such a patient can be recognized by the fact that the leg on the affected side is stiff and swings outward and forwards in a circular fashion rather than being lifted from the ground. In such patients the upper limb is often flexed at the elbow and adducted across the chest and is rarely moved.

Galactosaemia

The sign of a disease caused by an inborn error of metabolism in which the enzymes responsible for the breakdown of galactose, which is derived from milk, are deficient. The result is the accumulation of excessive quantities of galactose in the blood and tissues. This results in the development of DIARRHOEA, VOMITING, JAUNDICE, brain damage and hepatic enlargement (HEPATOMEGALY) in the affected infant. These undesirable consequences can be avoided if the condition is recognized at an early age and the baby is fed on a galactose-free diet. It is, however, difficult to avoid some damage particularly to the brain. Such dietary restriction must be continued throughout life.

Gall bladder colic

The classical pain of gall stones in which the patient complains of a relatively ill-localized epigastric pain which radiates to the tip of the right scapula. BILIARY COLIC is often accompanied by tenderness on pressure in the right subcostal region particularly on deep inspiration, MURPHY'S SIGN.

If the gall stone passes from the gall bladder into the common bile duct it may remain silent or alternatively cause obstructive JAUNDICE. Should the stone remain impacted in the cystic duct an INFLAMMATION of the gall bladder develops causing acute cholecystitis.

See COLIC and BILIARY COLIC.

Gangrene

Most commonly gangrene, or massive tissue necrosis, is a sign of a deficient blood flow to the tissues although occasionally it results from infection of the tissues with putrefactive organisms such as the anaerobic clostridia or the bacteroides.

When due to deficient blood flow and therefore a lack of oxygen to the tissues the affected part usually changes from blue to black and if the part is kept free from infection, a line, known as the line of demarcation, may develop between the dead and living tissues.

The onset of gangrene in the lower limb may be gradual and preceded by long history of intermittent CLAUDICATION if the arteries supplying the affected part are gradually occluded, or it may be sudden if the blood supply is suddenly brought to a halt.

The common causes of gangrene include:

(1) Atherosclerosis. In this condition the gradual deposition of fatty materials in the wall of medium-sized arteries such as the femoral, popliteal or coronary blood vessels causes a slowly decreasing flow of blood to the affected part. In the limbs the onset of gangrene is, therefore, preceded by a long history of intermittent claudication, whilst in the heart a myocardial infarction may be preceded by ANGINA pectoris.

As atherosclerosis progresses the intimal wall of

91

the artery becomes involved and eventually destroyed with the result that there are two possible complications of this disease which may lead to a rapid cessation of blood flow and thus precipitate the acute onset of gangrene:

(a) Thrombosis. The accumulation of platelets and the constituents of the blood such as red cells and fibrinogen in the form of a thrombus may cause acute occlusion.

(b) Embolus. An embolus in this instance is part of a thrombus which has broken loose and is carried along the artery until it can pass no further. At this point the embolus impacts and brings the circulation to a halt. The ultimate effect of such an embolus depends upon:

  (i) The size of the blood vessel it has blocked.
  (ii) The presence of collateral vessels which may be able to bypass the blocked segment.
  (iii) The tissue involved.

(2) Extrinsic pressure on the arterial supply, for example, in the limbs. A fracture of the tibia may occasionally be associated with such a degree of soft tissue swelling within the fascial compartments that the arterial supply to the foot is occluded. A similar effect may of course be caused by swelling of the limb within a too tight plaster cast or bandage and rarely by the over-long application of a tourniquet.

A similar mechanism is also involved in strangulation of the intestinal tract which is most commonly caused by external pressure on the mesenteric arteries and veins as in a strangulated external or internal hernia.

(3) Vasospastic disease, for example Raynaud's disease. This is the only common cause of gangrene in the upper limb. The vasospasm is usually precipitated by cold or emotional upset. The fingers go white, later blue and finally red during the recovery period. In severe cases gangrene of the fingertips occurs. Similar vasospastic changes may follow the prolonged use of pneumatic

drills, accidental poisoning with ergot or systemic sclerosis.

(4) Actual injury to an artery. The artery may be severed by a knife wound or the wall merely bruised whereupon thrombosis follows. The latter occurs in association with fractures, e.g. injury to the brachial artery following a fracture of the humerus or fracture dislocations, e.g. injury to the popliteal artery following dislocation of the knee joint.

Gigantism

An increase in height caused by an overgrowth of the skeleton. The underlying cause is an over-secretion of growth hormone by the cells of the anterior hypophysis (pituitary gland) prior to the fusion of the epiphyses which occurs at the age of 16 years in girls and 18 years in boys.

Once fusion of the epiphyses has occurred, a similar over-secretion of growth hormone, caused usually by an adenoma of the anterior part of the hypophysis, causes the disease known as ACROMEGALY in which one of the first and most significant features is a change in the facial appearance due to thickening of the skin and underlying subcutaneous tissues. The skull may enlarge and the lower jaw protrude, changes caused by overgrowth of these bones which are formed in membrane and not cartilage.

Glycosuria

Normal urine usually contains very little, if any, sugar. If sufficient is present to be detected by simple tests such as the Clinitest or Benedict's test, the condition of glycosuria is present.

The reason that there is little or no sugar in a normal urine is because glucose, which passes from the blood stream through the renal glomeruli into the tubules of the nephron, is normally reabsorbed into the blood. However, when the blood sugar exceeds 10 mmol/litre, more sugar is filtered through the glomeruli into the tubules than can be reabsorbed and so sugar appears in the urine.

The 2 common causes of glycosuria are:

(1) Renal glycosuria. This is a harmless hereditary condition which occurs in approximately 5 in 10 000 persons. In this condition the capacity of tubules to absorb glucose is less than normal and as a result, at much lower blood sugar levels glucose appears in the urine.

(2) Diabetes mellitus. In this relatively common disease, affecting about one per cent of the population of Great Britain, the secretion of the hormone insulin by the islet cells of the pancreas, or the effectiveness of the hormone, is abolished or diminished. Glucose metabolism is impaired and the blood sugar rises. Since increasing quantities of glucose are now filtered through the glomeruli, glycosuria occurs. Excessive glucose in the tubules attracts water by its osmotic effect, with the result that polyuria occurs. The loss of water in turn leads to an increased thirst, which is one of the common presenting symptoms of diabetes.

Goitre

A swelling of the neck due to enlargement of the thyroid gland which may involve either a part or a whole of the organ.

Enlargement of the whole gland is usually due to:

(1) Deficiency of iodine in the diet which causes swelling of the gland due to hyperplasia and later the accumulation of colloid in the follicles of the gland. The latter is often known as a colloid goitre. In middle age such glands lose their smooth outline and become nodular. Simple goitre is not associated with hormonal disturbance.

(2) Primary thyrotoxicosis. This type of goitre is associated with thyrotoxicosis.

(3) Hashimoto's disease, or lymphadenoid goitre. This goitre is associated with myxoedema.

(4) Cancer of the thyroid.

A local enlargement of the gland may be caused by:

(1) The development of false 'adenoma' in a gland already the seat of a simple iodine deficiency goitre.

(2) A true benign tumour of the gland. This is relatively rare.

(3) Some forms of cancer of the thyroid.

Aside from any hormonal effects a goitre may cause physical symptoms compressing the trachea causing STRIDOR, or the oesophagus causing DYSPHAGIA. Alternatively, if the lower pole of the enlarging gland grows down behind the sternum, the trachea may only be compressed when the neck is in certain positions, as for example in bed at night. This may cause the patient to wake up gasping for breath due to the sudden onset of respiratory obstruction. Cancer of the thyroid may also invade or compress the recurrent laryngeal nerves which lie in the neck to such an extent that the vocal cord on the affected side is paralysed causing hoarseness of the voice.

Gradenigo's syndrome

A syndrome occasionally seen in patients suffering from acute INFLAMMATION of the mastoid (mastoiditis); it consists of an inability to rotate the eye on the affected side in a lateral direction. The presence of this sign indicates that the infection has spread from the mastoid to the petrous portion of the temporal bone because only in this area can the 6th cranial nerve, which supplies the muscle involved in lateral rotation be damaged.

Gynaecomastia

Enlargement of the male breast. Unilateral or bilateral gynaecomastia may be seen in normal adolescent boys and also at the age of the male menopause, either may prove an embarrassment to the affected individual. The cause of this type of enlargement is usually ascribed to hormonal variation.

Bilateral gynaecomastia may also be a sign of the following disorders:

(1) Chronic liver failure due to advanced cirrhosis in which the liver is unable to detoxify the oestrogenic hormones which flow through it. At the same time the testes undergo ATROPHY. In such individuals there are usually other signs of chronic liver failure, HEPATOMEGALY, CAPUT MEDUSAE and possibly, HEPATIC ENCEPHALO-PATHY.

(2) Oestrogen-producing tumours of the testicle. These are

rare but if arising in the interstitial cells may produce sufficient oestrogen to cause enlargement of the breasts.

Unilateral enlargement of the male breast is rarely due to carcinoma. However in such patients the obvious signs of cancer may be found; enlargement of the breast, fixity of the underlying mass to both skin and deeper structures, retraction of the nipple and possibly the presence of lymphatic metastases.

Haematemesis

The VOMITING of blood. Depending upon the site from which the bleeding occurs, the volume and the length of time the blood has remained in the stomach, if at all, the vomit may vary in colour—from the red colour, associated with pure blood, to a brownish colour, due to the change by the gastric juice of the haemoglobin to acid haematin (COFFEE-GROUND VOMIT). The patient may FAINT following a haematemesis, or, with the loss of larger volumes, develop SHOCK.

The causes of haematemesis are numerous. Blood may be swallowed and then vomited. This is particularly common following a severe nose bleed. More commonly the cause of a haematemesis lies in a pathological condition affecting:

(1) The oesophagus.
(2) The stomach or duodenum.
(3) The blood, e.g. PURPURA or leukaemia.

In addition there are a large number of miscellaneous causes which include prolonged JAUNDICE, abdominal injury and perforation of an aneurysm into the stomach.

Haematemesis occurs most frequently in association with the following:

(1) Erosions of the gastric mucosa which may follow the excessive ingestion of alcohol or the taking of aspirin.
(2) Chronic duodenal ULCERATION.
(3) Chronic gastric ulceration.
(4) Oesophageal varices in patients suffering from portal HYPERTENSION due to cirrhosis of the liver.
(5) Gastric tumours.
(6) Tears of the oesophageal mucosa due to vomiting.

In about 50 per cent of patients the source of the bleeding may be decided from the clinical history and the physical signs of disease alone, but in the remaining patients the source can only be determined following investigations which include:

(1) Oesophagoscopy, gastroscopy and duodenoscopy.
(2) Radiological investigation by barium swallow and meal.

It is important to establish the cause of the bleeding as quickly as possible so that the management of the patient may be planned. This may be by medical means or by surgery. The latter would be indicated, for example, in patients suffering from chronic duodenal ulceration in whom repeated bleeding had occurred, whereas acute gastric erosions usually respond to medical treatment provided that the blood lost is replaced.

Haematoma

A collection of blood in the tissues usually caused by accidental or deliberate injury, the magnitude of the haematoma being commonly related to the severity of the injury.

However, in conditions such as HAEMOPHILIA in which there is a defect in the mechanisms responsible for the coagulation of blood, haematomata, especially in the muscles, may develop after relatively trivial injuries and form one of the major complications of the disease.

When a haematoma develops in the subcutaneous tissues the haemoglobin liberated from the erythrocytes is slowly broken down by the tissue enzymes causing a characteristic series of colour changes in the skin, commonly known as bruising.

The overall importance of haematoma depends upon:

(1) Its size, a large haematoma may cause ANAEMIA.
(2) Its position, a haematoma developing in the subdural space following a head injury attracts fluid and by slowly enlarging may mimic the signs and symptoms of a brain tumour, the patient developing HEADACHES, drowsiness and mental confusion together with PAPILLOEDEMA and a variety of signs involving the nervous system.
(3) The development of complications, the commonest of which is infection since blood provides an ideal medium for the growth of bacteria.

Haematuria

The passage of red blood cells in the urine. Rapid tests to confirm the presence of haemoglobin in the urine are now available. These are necessary because a reddish urine may result from the excretion of pigment present in beetroot, senna and some proprietary purgatives which contain the indicator phenophthalein which turns red in an alkaline urine. The Haemostix, commonly used, is a strip impregnated with a chemical substance known as orthotolidine. Dipped into urine, a blue colour appearing within 30 seconds indicates the presence of blood. However, to distinguish between HAEMOGLOBINURIA and haematuria the urine must be examined under a microscope to detect the presence of intact erythrocytes.

The source of the bleeding is often suggested by the colour of the urine, thus a 'smoky' urine indicates that the blood is intimately mixed with the urine and that the probable source is the kidney whereas a 'port wine' stained urine or a urine containing clots suggests that the blood is originating in the bladder, commonly from a tumour, less commonly from severe INFLAMMATION.

Haematuria may result from general conditions or it may result from diseases of the urinary tract.

General conditions leading to haematuria include:

(1) Malignant HYPERTENSION.
(2) Thrombocytopenic PURPURA, primary or secondary, in which there is a reduction in the number of platelets.

Local conditions of the renal tract include:

(1) Tumours, benign or malignant of the kidney, ureter or bladder.
(2) Acute and chronic infections of the urinary tract, including acute pyelonephritis and acute cystitis, tuberculosis and schistosomiasis.
(3) Stones.
(4) Injury to any part of the tract.
(5) Senile enlargement of the prostate.
(6) Acute glomerulo-nephritis.

Haemoglobinuria

A brown or black discolouration of the urine due to the presence of haemoglobin.

Haemoglobinuria can only follow massive and explosive intravascular haemolysis, i.e. the breakdown of red cells, because under normal conditions the haemoglobin liberated from red cells is converted to bilirubin.

Such rapid breakdown occurs as a result of:

(1) An incompatible blood transfusion when the incompatible donor cells are immediately destroyed.

(2) Extensive burns when the erythrocytes flowing through the capillaries, arterioles or arteries are damaged by the thermal injury in the area of the burn or scald.

(3) Severe specific infections including:

    (a) Gas GANGRENE in which the responsible anaerobic bacteria known as the clostridia produce exotoxins which break down the erythrocytes.

    (b) Yellow fever, an acute virus infection transmitted by the mosquito, commonest in Africa. In severe disease the affected person dies within 5 to 6 days.

(4) Certain drugs such as phenylhydrazine, once used in the treatment of polycythaemia.

Haemophilia

This condition is a sign of a deficiency of clotting Factor VIII in the blood. It is inherited by a sex-linked recessive gene so that although the female carries the defective gene she very rarely shows evidence of the disease.

The usual symptom of haemophilia is a tendency to bleed, either spontaneously or following minor trauma, into the deeper tissues or joints. Spontaneous HAEMATURIA and nose bleeding can also occur but these patients usually do not suffer from spontaneous capillary bleeding unlike sufferers from capillary disorders such as von Willebrand's disease.

The ease with which bleeding is precipitated in haemophilia is largely determined by the level of circulating Factor VIII which varies considerably in different patients. Repeated attacks of bleeding into joints or soft tissues may eventually cause gross disablement due to organization of the resulting clot producing intra-articular adhesions, erosion of the articular cartilage and fibrous bands within the muscles. When a severe haemophiliac requires an operation the deficiency of the clotting factor must be corrected for at least twelve days after the operation by the administration of antihaemophilic globulin.

Haemoptysis

The coughing up of blood in the form of a frothy blood-stained sputum or as small clots. If the blood is coughed up immediately it will be bright red, but if there is any delay the oxyhaemoglobin is reduced and the sputum then appears darker or 'rust' coloured.

The chief causes of haemoptysis include:

(1) Left ventricular HEART FAILURE due to mitral stenosis. In this condition the bleeding arises from the congested capillaries which surround the alveoli.

(2) Pulmonary infarction. This condition follows prolonged immobilization in bed or more commonly, a surgical operation. This infarct is caused by a clot formed in and dislodged from the pelvic veins or the deep veins of the leg. The clot impacts in the lumen of the pulmonary artery or its branches and due to the extreme vascularity of lung tissue and also its laxity, intense engorgement of the affected area follows. The over-distended capillaries rupture and haemoptysis follows.

(3) Inflammation of the lungs or disease of the bronchi, including:

(a) Tuberculosis, due to ULCERATION of the air passages or erosion of blood vessels.

(b) Lobar pneumonia, due to the congestion of the alveoli with red blood cells.

(c) Bronchiectasis, due to ulceration of air passage.

(4) Tumours of the lung, malignant or benign.

Haemorrhage

Haemorrhage or bleeding is the escape of blood from a blood vessel. It may be classified in various ways:

(1) According to the type of vessel involved:
   (a) Arterial.
   (b) Capillary.
   (c) Venous.

(2) According to the time of occurrence:
   (a) Primary, occurring at the time of injury or surgery.
   (b) Reactionary, occurring within 24 to 48 hours of the injury or the operation. Reactionary haemorrhage occurs due to the displacement of an insecure ligature or clot.
   (c) Secondary, occurring 7 to 10 days after injury or surgery when infection has eroded the wall of the blood vessel and the contained thrombus.

(3) According to the site:
   (a) External haemorrhage indicates that blood can be seen leaving the body.
   (b) Internal haemorrhage is bleeding into the interior of a cavity such as the skull, chest or the tissues.

(4) According to cause: in the majority of patients suffering from a haemorrhage the cause is simple trauma, but in a minority there is some underlying pathological process which may include:
   (a) HYPERTENSION, uncontrollable EPISTAXIS may be the first presenting symptom of this condition.
   (b) A reduction in the number of platelets in the blood, THROMBOCYTOPENIA. Platelet deficiencies from any cause are usually associated with petechial haemorrhages or purpuric rashes.
   (c) A deficiency in the coagulation mechanisms. The classic condition associated with a coagulation defect is HAEMOPHILIA, often first discovered when unexpectedly severe bleeding takes place into a joint or the tissues following a minor injury. A somewhat commoner cause of defective coagulation is severe

liver disease due to the inability of a damaged liver to manufacture the various coagulation factors, one of the most important of which is fibrinogen.

Physiological response to injury: Damage to a blood vessel is followed by a series of changes all of which occur in an attempt by nature to prevent excessive haemorrhage. First, the injured vessel contracts; second, platelets adhere to the damaged endothelium liberating a variety of enzymes which initiate the clotting process. These responses may be quite enough to deal with the damage to smaller blood vessels, but when a large artery or vein is involved, surgical treatment in the form of ligature may be required in order to prevent death from haemorrhagic SHOCK. In some sites such as within the skull, an internal haemorrhage is dangerous not because of its volume but because of the destruction of nervous tissue which occurs, and the increasing INTRACRANIAL PRESSURE.

Hallucination

The perception of sensory stimuli which do not exist in reality. The hallucinating patient sees or hears something although there is nothing to see or hear.

Hallucinations, which may involve any of the sensory systems, visual, auditory, touch or smell, are a characteristic feature of disordered brain function and occur in a variety of diseases including:

(1) Drug-induced disorders such as alcoholism or barbiturate poisoning.
(2) Severe infections such as meningitis or cerebral malaria.
(3) SEPTICAEMIA.
(4) Severely anoxic patients, or patients suffering from respiratory ACIDOSIS.
(5) (a) Depression, the depressed individual occasionally hears auditory hallucinations which are nearly always 'accusative'.
    (b) Schizophrenia. In this mental disorder visual hallucinations are commonplace.

Headache

A headache is a symptom occurring in many different conditions and it is of particular importance when attempting to establish the cause to ascertain the site, quality, intensity, radiation, precipitating factors and the presence or absence of any accompanying symptoms.

The common causes of headaches include:

(1) Functional conditions such as ANXIETY, HYSTERIA and depression.

(2) Conditions associated with alterations in the cerebral blood flow such as migraine and HYPERTENSION.

(3) Metabolic disturbances such as HYPOGLYCAEMIA.

(4) Conditions causing an increase in the INTRACRANIAL PRESSURE such as primary or secondary neoplasms, ABSCESSES and extradural, subdural or intracerebral HAEMATOMA which may follow a head injury. The headache associated with a gradual increase in the intracranial pressure usually possesses certain characteristic features. The patient tends to wake with a throbbing headache affecting the temporal regions and usually complains of VOMITING but no NAUSEA. As the day progresses the symptoms often improve but unfortunately they recur each morning with increasing severity until drowsiness and COMA supervene. In addition the symptoms and signs of damage to nervous tissue occur such as HEMIANOPIA or ATAXIA. Such signs are often helpful in deciding the site of the developing tumour within the brain.

(5) Disease of the meninges which cover the brain including subarachnoid HAEMORRHAGE and bacterial or viral meningitis.

(6) Injuries to the head leading to CONCUSSION or CONTUSIONS or lacerations of the brain tissue.

(7) Headache may be a REFERRED PAIN from disease involving other structures such as sinusitis, acute glaucoma or temporal arteritis.

Heart block

Heart block is the most important cardiac cause of BRADY-CARDIA and is commonly the result of ischaemic heart disease or the toxic effect of drugs which act upon the heart such as digitalis and its derivatives.

In heart block, from whatever cause, the impulses which normally stimulate contraction of the ventricular muscle fail to reach it with the result that the rate of ventricular contraction, and hence of the peripheral pulse, slows appreciably.

Even in complete heart block the rate of ventricular contraction falls only to 30 to 40 beats per minute because the muscles of the ventricle possess their own inherent property of spontaneous rhythmic contraction regardless of external influences. A heart rate of this speed provides a blood flow adequate for the body's needs at rest, but vigorous exercise becomes impossible because the heart rate cannot increase in order to supply the increased demand for blood by the active tissues. In partial heart block the difference between the rate of atrial and ventricular contraction is considerably less although the condition can be readily recognized by electrocardiography.

Heart failure

A sign that a diseased heart is unable to maintain a cardiac output sufficient for the needs of the body.

When the loss of cardiac efficiency occurs suddenly the patient develops cardiogenic SHOCK, a situation frequently seen after a massive coronary thrombosis which produces a large myocardial infarction.

More commonly the heart fails gradually, frequently with the initial emphasis falling on the right or left side each of which produces its own specific symptoms and signs.

Right-sided failure occurs when the right ventricle can no longer pump blood to the lungs for oxygenation. The common causes are chronic lung disease and mitral stenosis, the presence of either increasing the work load of the right ventricle. At the point at which the right ventricle fails back pressure develops in the systemic venous system via the right atrium and the superior and inferior vena cavae. The result is usually

OEDEMA particularly of the lower limbs or dependent areas. Thus a patient confined to bed develops oedema over the sacrum. In addition the liver becomes engorged, one of the factors leading to ASCITES. The jugular veins become congested (see JUGULAR VEIN ENGORGEMENT) and can be observed pulsating with each cardiac contraction.

Left-sided heart failure results in the retention of blood in the lungs, the capillaries of which become congested leading to pulmonary OEDEMA and attacks of CARDIAC ASTHMA. Failure of the left side of the heart eventually affects the right side causing congestive heart failure. The common causes of left-sided failure include HYPERTENSION, disease of the aortic valves producing narrowing of the outlet, and ischaemic heart disease.

Heartburn

A retrosternal burning pain which may occasionally occur in a perfectly normal individual but if persistent usually indicates an oesophageal disorder.

The commonest cause of this symptom is the regurgitation of acid from the stomach into the oesophagus which, if persistent, causes an inflammation of this viscus. In a normal individual, such regurgitation is uncommon but in conditions such as hiatus hernia, the mechanisms preventing the escape of gastric contents through the junction between oesophagus and stomach are disorganized. The symptom is usually made worse by activities which lead to an increase in the intra-abdominal pressure such as stooping or lying down. Naturally occurring conditions such as pregnancy may be associated with severe heartburn.

A similar sensation may also be produced by excessively active contractions of the oesophagus in which condition there need not necessarily be any abnormality of the lining of the oesophagus.

Heberden's nodules

Swellings about the size of a pea developing over the dorsum of the terminal interphalangeal joints. The swellings are composed of bony or cartilaginous outgrowths from the phalanges and are often accompanied by an outpouching of the synovial membrane of the joint, so that a considerable deformity is eventually caused.

Heberden's nodes are a sign of osteoarthrosis and tend to show a high familial incidence, especially in the female members of a family.

Hemianopia

A form of blindness in which only a part of the visual fields is affected.

Hemianopia is usually a sign of damage to the optic chiasma or the nerve tracts within the brain known as the optic radiations. The optic chiasma which is situated at the base of the brain is the name given to the point at which the optic nerves meet. In the chiasma the fibres from the lateral parts of the visual fields pass onwards into the same side of the brain, whereas the optic nerve fibres from the inner field of the eye cross over to enter the opposite half of the brain.

The common cause of derangement of the optic chiasma is the presence of a tumour of the hypophysis or hypothalamus. Either may compress or invade the chiasma and the first part to be affected is usually the central portion containing the fibres which cross over and so the temporal fields of vision are disturbed or destroyed. This is known as bitemporal hemianopia because the outer part of the visual fields of both eyes is disturbed.

Lesions of the brain itself such as tumours growing in and affecting the optic radiations themselves cause a homonymous hemianopia in which the same side of the visual field is lost in both eyes because of the damage done to fibres which have already crossed over in the chiasma.

Hemiplegia see STROKE

A condition in which there is PARALYSIS of one half of the body due to disease of the upper, as opposed to the lower, motor neurone.

Hemiplegia is usually the result of an intracranial disease, although very occasionally it can be the result of a lesion in the high cervical cord in which event there is no paralysis of the face.

Henoch–Schoenlein syndrome

Also known as anaphylactoid PURPURA or allergic purpura. A condition probably caused by a hypersensitivity reaction which, by damaging the small blood vessels, increases their permeability and allows an exudation of erythrocytes and plasma to occur into surrounding tissues. This causes purpura, OEDEMA and URTICARIA.

The syndrome usually affects children and young adults and a typical attack usually occurs within one to 4 weeks of an acute respiratory tract infection. The classical symptoms, all of which arise from the various sites of bleeding, are ABDOMINAL AND JOINT PAINS, together with a PURPURIC skin rash.

Hepatic encephalopathy

A sign of acute or chronic disease of the liver caused by the effect on the brain of, as yet, unidentified chemical substances which would normally be detoxified by the liver.

The symptoms of acute encephalophathy include listlessness, drowsiness, incoherence and DELIRIUM. Later COMA develops with increased tendon reflexes and a positive BABINSKI SIGN. Muscle twitching, OPISTHOTONOS and CONVULSIONS occur. When the cause is a fulminating viral hepatitis these symptoms and signs may precede the appearance of JAUNDICE by as much as 48 hours.

Chronic hepatic encephalopathy is dominated by the symptoms of cerebral and cerebellar disease. In some patients a progressive loss of intellect occurs, in others alternating excitement and apathy and in yet others HALLUCINATIONS and DELUSIONS. In addition a characteristic TREMOR develops somewhat similar to that seen in PARKINSONISM, at its worst the tremor is flapping in character, coarse movements taking place at the wrist and metacarpophalangeal joints. ATHETOSIS may occur and the speech is often slurred and very indistinct.

Hepatomegaly

The commoner causes of enlargement of the liver include:
  (1) Acute infections including viral hepatitis, malaria, hepatic ABSCESS.

107

(2) Chronic infections including tuberculosis, syphilis and actinomycosis.

(3) Cirrhosis.

(4) Malignant disease:

(a) Primary tumours which are very rare.

(b) Secondary metastases which are very common.

(5) Diseases of the lymphoid tissues including Hodgkin's disease.

(6) HEART FAILURE.

Hepatomegaly like SPLENOMEGALY rarely causes symptoms although the weight of a greatly enlarged liver may occasionally produce a sensation of discomfort in the upper abdomen. Infective conditions producing rapid enlargement and stretching of the liver capsule may cause considerable discomfort. Abscesses, from whatever cause, are associated with both PAIN and FEVER but in the majority of patients suffering from hepatomegaly the symptoms are those of the underlying disease.

Hermaphroditism

A condition in which both ovarian and testicular tissue are present in the same individual. Nearly all hermaphrodites suffer from an enlarged clitoris suggesting that they are male. Close examination may reveal an apparently total hypospadias and what appears to be a vaginal orifice, the scrotum will be improperly formed and lie, somewhat like enlarged labia majora on either side of the median opening. Any swellings detected in these folds will probably be testicular. Laparotomy reveals uterus, tubes and ovaries. A decision has to be made at an early date as to the sex in which the child is to be reared. Once this decision has been made surgical correction of the various anatomical faults is required.

Hiccup

A type of COUGH produced by a sudden contraction of the diaphragm after the glottis has been closed by adduction of the vocal cords. The diaphragmatic contractions are most commonly intermittent, but may be so persistent that the patient becomes physically exhausted.

Hiccups occur in perfectly normal individuals sometimes after eating hot peppery foods, over-indulgence of alcohol or they may also occur in physically healthy HYSTERICS.

The organic causes which may be associated with hiccuping include:

(1) Diaphragmatic irritation: From above this may be caused by pneumonia causing diaphragmatic pleurisy, from below the diaphragm may be irritated by peritonitis.

(2) Local conditions in the brain affecting that area from which the phrenic nerve takes origin. Thus, hiccuping may occur when a vascular lesion or a tumour affects this part of the base of the brain, or an inflammatory condition such as encephalitis.

(3) General conditions: Hiccuping is not uncommon in uraemia.

High-stepping gait

The type of gait observed in patients suffering from foot-drop in which the dorsiflexors of the foot are paralysed. As a result the patient flexes the hip and knee in an exaggerated fashion in order to avoid dragging the toes along the ground when walking.

Hirsutism

The excessive growth of hair of male distribution in a female. Mild excesses are commonplace, said to affect between 10 to 30 per cent of young caucasian women in the absence of any endocrine disorder or menstrual irregularity. In many such women there is a family history or the condition may be related to race, thus women of Mediterranean extraction are hairier than are Europeans. In many of these women slightly abnormal blood levels of androgenic steroids can be demonstrated even though they demonstrate no evidence of VIRILISM in the form of clitoral hypertrophy, deepening of the voice or menstrual irregularity.

Other than this group of women, all other causes of hirsutism are rare and include:

(1) Iatrogenic causes. The administration of testosterone or

a pure anabolic steroid to a woman will certainly cause hirsutism. In some patients receiving the drug deca-durabolin hirsutism occurs and lastly, excessive doses of cortisone may be followed by marked hirsutism.

(2) Cushing's disease or syndrome. The former caused by a tumour of the anterior hypophysis and the latter by hyperplasia, adenoma or tumour of the adrenal cortex. In addition to HIRSUTISM the sufferers from this disease become OBESE, develop weakness of the skeletal muscles, easy bruising due to fragility of the capillary walls and deformities of the spine due to osteoporosis. Occasionally, in addition to hirsutism an element of VIRILISM occurs.

(3) Polycystic ovarian syndrome, otherwise known as the Stein–Leventhalsyndrome. In this condition the sufferers develop hirsutism and obesity, together with oligomenorrhoea or AMENORRHOEA. The ovaries are enlarged, cystic and have thickened fibrous capsules. Investigation of the various hormonal changes in this syndrome shows that there is a disproportionate production of androgens.

(4) Congenital adrenal hyperplasia, see Virilism.

Horner's syndrome

A condition produced by damage to the cervical sympathetic nervous system in which:

(1) The pupil of the eye is constricted because of the unopposed action of the parasympathetic nerve supply.

(2) The upper eyelid is lower than on the normal unaffected side because the muscle involved, the levator palpebrae superioris, is paralysed.

(3) There is anhydrosis, or absence of sweating on the affected side.

This condition may follow sympathectomy, injury to the brachial plexus or invasion of the sympathetic trunk by malignant disease.

Hunger pain

A sensation of epigastric discomfort which may occur in a perfectly normal healthy but hungry individual, possibly arising from spasm of the smooth muscle of the stomach and duodenum.

Hunger also precipitates severe epigastric pain in patients suffering from duodenal ULCERATION usually some hours after a normal meal or between 2 and 3 a.m. The cause is the gastric hydrochloric acid in contact with the ulcerated area stimulating the exposed nerve endings in the base of the ulcer. In addition to causing visceral pain, spasm of the pyloric muscle also occurs so that VOMITING is an added feature.

In carcinoma of the stomach such pain rarely occurs because no acid is present in the condition.

Hyperchondriasis

A symptom associated with ANXIETY in which an individual is affected by morbid apprehensions about the state of his/her health. The patient usually develops a number of symptoms, all with a FUNCTIONAL basis. Seeking medical advice, the affected individual fails to be convinced of the true explanation of the symptoms and so travels from doctor to doctor always seeking relief but never finding it.

Hyperhydrosis

Excessive sweating which may occur in normal individuals, in response to emotional stress or adverse environmental conditions, and in some apparently normal individuals such disabling sweating of the hands and feet may occur that it can only be controlled by the operation of sympathectomy.

Pathological conditions associated with hyperhydrosis include:

(1) Thyrotoxicosis and tumours of the adrenal medulla known as phaeochromocytoma. In both these disorders the autonomic nervous system which controls the sweat glands is deranged and in addition the metabolic rate is increased necessitating an increase in heat loss from the body.

111

(2) In some individuals hyperhydrosis only affects the particular sweat glands of the axilla, perineum and groins. If infection occurs this leads to the clinical condition known as hyperhydrosis suppurativa, an unpleasant condition which is difficult to cure without the total excision of the skin of the affected areas.

Hyper-pigmentation

A generalized increase in the pigmentation of the skin caused by an accumulation of melanin is a sign of Addison's disease in which the adrenal cortex is destroyed by disease. As a result a compensatory increase occurs in the hormonal secretion of the hypophysis cerebri, a part of which acts to stimulate melanin production.

This hyper-pigmentation is most marked in the skin creases and around the nipples and perineum. Careful inspection of the mouth also reveals patches of pigment, typically on the buccal mucosa close to the molar teeth.

When hyper-pigmentation is related to Addison's disease there are many associated symptoms and signs including anorexia, HYPOGLYCAEMIA, apathy and a lowered blood pressure, due to absence of the main adrenal hormone cortisol which controls the distribution of salt and water in the tissues.

Similar pigmentation may be seen in arsenical poisoning, chronic liver disease, malignant CACHEXIA and pellagra, but in all these conditions the mucous membranes are seldom affected.

Hyperpyrexia

A life-threatening rise in body temperature to above 41°C. Such high temperatures can only develop when the heat-regulating centre at the base of the brain has broken down with the result that the physiological processes by which the body loses heat do not occur.

Hyperpyrexia can develop in perfectly normal individuals when exposed to high environmental temperatures or performing excessive muscular activity. The body normally loses heat by evaporation, convection and conduction but in the tropics heat loss by these means is greatly reduced leading to the clini-

112

cal condition of 'heat stroke' in which the affected individual not only develops hyperpyrexia but also CONVULSIONS, COMA and damage to the kidneys.

Diseases associated with hyperpyrexia include:

(1) A rare condition known as congenital ectodermal dysplasia in which the sweat glands are defective. This reduces the ability to sweat and, therefore, to lose heat by evaporation.

(2) Infection. Hyperpyrexia is particularly common when the brain and meninges are involved as in meningococcal meningitis and cerebral malaria although it can also occur in other infections.

(3) Severe head injuries in which damage has occurred in an area of the brain known as the pons which is close to the heat-regulating centre.

(4) Thyroid CRISIS, a condition usually seen in thyrotoxic patients improperly prepared for the operation of thyroidectomy. Occasionally, however, thyrotoxicosis may go unrecognized and an operation performed on such a patient or the development of intercurrent infection may then precipitate such a crisis. Both the pulse and temperature rise rapidly, the patient becomes confused and DELIRIOUS and finally, untreated, passes into COMA.

(5) On very rare occasions hyperpyrexia follows general anaesthesia usually involving the use of relaxant drugs.

Hypertension

An abnormal elevation of the blood pressure. Hypertension may occur in perfectly normal individuals due to fear or ANXIETY, physical exercise or smoking and before, therefore, an individual is considered to be hypertensive, the blood pressure must be repeatedly measured, if possible, in conditions of emotional and physical rest.

Hypertension is often classified as benign or malignant. Malignant hypertension is associated with:

(1) A diastolic blood pressure of 120 mmHg or over.
(2) PAPILLOEDEMA.
(3) Pathological changes in the arterioles.

113

The causes of hypertension are:

(1) Idiopathic, often referred to as essential hypertension. In this group the cardiac output remains normal but the resistance to the flow of blood in the periphery of the circulation increases. Initially the arterioles are normal in appearance but as the condition progresses changes in their structure develop. Finally atherosclerosis occurs in the larger blood vessels. Myocardial hypertrophy accompanied by enlargement of the heart also develops due to the increasing work the heart must perform in order to pump blood into the resistant circulation. In malignant hypertension even greater changes in the arterioles occur particularly in the kidney and also in the brain and elsewhere. These changes associated with the higher blood pressure in this condition predispose to the development of acute attacks of cerebral symptoms including HEADACHE, NAUSEA, VOMITING, apathy and even epileptiform CONVULSIONS, together with the presence of PROTEINURIA. In a normal individual the development of sudden hypertension due, for example, to an emotional crisis brings reflex mechanisms into play which operate through sensors in the great vessels. These bring the blood pressure back to normal within a reasonable time. In essential hypertension these same reflexes appear to be abolished.

(2) Secondary hypertension occurs in the presence of pre-existing disease:
   (a) Diseases affecting the kidney, e.g. glomerulo-nephritis.
   (b) Endocrine disorders:
      (i) Tumours of the hypophysis causing Cushing's disease or ACROMEGALY.
      (ii) Tumours of the adrenal gland which may be of the medulla, phaeochromocytoma or of the cortex, producing CUSHING'S SYNDROME or primary aldosteronism.
   (c) Coarctation of the aorta.
   (d) Hypertension associated with pregnancy.
   (e) Acute lead poisoning.

In the majority of individuals hypertension is discovered on routine examination during examinations for insurance or superannuation purposes. If symptoms occur they are usually the result of complications affecting the heart e.g. HEART FAILURE, the brain e.g. headache, or STROKE, or the kidneys e.g. POLYURIA associated with albumin in the urine.

Hyperthyroidism

A symptom complex associated with the excessive production of thyroid hormone by the thyroid gland, although occasionally it may follow the over-administration of this hormone in patients suffering from HYPOTHYROIDISM.

Since the thyroid hormone governs the overall rate of cellular metabolism, the symptoms and signs of its over-secretion affect nearly all the systems of the body.

Thus in consequence of the overall increase in metabolism there is an increase in heat production with the result that the skin is warm, flushed and moist through excessive sweating. The appetite increases but usually not sufficiently to compensate for the increased energy expenditure and therefore the patient loses weight.

Tachycardia develops, and in long-standing untreated cases, there may be ATRIAL FIBRILLATION. DIARRHOEA may occur. The various eye signs such as LID LAG and EXOPHTHALMOS are commonplace in the type of thyrotoxicosis occurring in young people, often known as Graves' disease or exophthalmic goitre to distinguish it from the disease as seen in older women which is usually preceded by a GOITRE of many years' standing.

Hypoglycaemia

A fall in the blood sugar concentration sufficient to cause symptoms and signs. The critical blood sugar level is about 50 mg/100 ml or 2.8 mmol/litre blood.

The development of symptoms depends on the absolute concentration of the circulating glucose and on the rate at which this concentration is reached. The commonest cause of hypoglycaemia is an overdose of insulin.

115

The less common causes include:

(1) Organic diseases, for example, HYPOTHYROIDISM, severe liver disease and insulin-producing tumours of the islet cell of the pancreas.
(2) Inborn errors of metabolism such as GALACTOSAEMIA.
(3) Reactive hypoglycaemia, as occurs following partial gastrectomy or gastro-jejunostomy.
(4) Excessive administration of drugs such as the salicylates or paracetamol.

The symptoms of hypoglycaemia are primarily due to the disturbed function of the nervous system which cannot operate properly in the absence of glucose which is its only source of energy.

A rapid fall in the circulating level of glucose causes nervousness, trembling, PALPITATION, sweating, twitching, unconsciousness and if very severe, death. Many of these symptoms are caused by the hormone, adrenaline, which is excreted in large amounts in response to hypoglycaemia.

When the concentration of glucose falls slowly the behaviour of the individual may resemble mild alcoholic intoxication with FUNCTIONAL impairment exceeding the subjective symptoms so that the patient is unable to appreciate the seriousness of his condition.

Hypopituitarism

A sign of deficiency in the circulating level of hormones produced by the hypophysis cerebri. This deficiency may occur rapidly due to infarction of the gland following a post-partum haemorrhage, SHEEHAN'S SYNDROME, or slowly due to the gradual growth of a tumour in the pituitary fossa causing Simmond's disease.

The affected individual complains of lack of energy, lack of libido, and if a woman, AMENORRHOEA. Depression and apathy are common. Weight is often maintained but occasionally the patient becomes CACHECTIC. The patient is pallid but not necessarily anaemic and the skin is pale and thin. A gradual loss of axillary and pubic hair takes place.

Hypothermia

A condition in which the normal body temperature cannot be maintained and the central or 'core' temperature falls.

A direct effect on the heart of excessive cooling is depression of the activity of the sino-atrial node leading to BRADYCARDIA followed by depression of the conducting system. This leads to varying degrees of HEART BLOCK and finally when the core temperature falls to about 30°C COMA develops followed by death from ventricular fibrillation.

The immediate response of the body to a cold environment is a reduction of the blood flow through the blood vessels of the skin and subcutaneous tissues by vasoconstriction in an attempt to conserve heat. This is followed by increasing the heat produced by the tissues either by voluntary movements, which are relatively inefficient, or by shivering.

A severe reduction in the body temperature may be caused by:

(1) Exposure to cold.

    (a) Hypothermia is a relatively common cause of death in the elderly or infirm. The gravity of the condition may not be recognized because an ordinary clinical thermometer does not register below 35°C.

    (b) Hypothermia is also a common cause of death following accidents at sea, a sea temperature approaching freezing is only compatible with survival for about one hour.

    (c) Hypothermia is a danger to every neonate because the baby lacks the intrinsic ability of the older child to maintain a constant body temperature.

(2) Prior to the development of adequate pump oxygenators hypothermia was deliberately induced in the anaesthetized patient in order to reduce the metabolism of the body. This enabled the surgeon to bring the circulation to a standstill for a period of up to 8 minutes without causing irreversible brain damage.

(3) The inadvertent transfusion of large quantities of blood, normally stored at 4°C, may lower the body temperature to such a degree that cardiac arrhythmias develop.

Hypothyroidism

A sign of insufficient thyroid hormone in the circulation the effects of which differ according to the age at which the deficiency occurs.

In the newborn child in whom the thyroid is either incompletely developed or totally absent cretinism occurs. The signs of this condition are failure of the infant to thrive and the rapid development of mental retardation. In addition the tongue enlarges causing obstruction of the nose and the symptoms of a persistent cold. Cretinism can only be prevented by early recognition and adequate replacement of the deficient hormone.

In the adult, hypothyroidism leads to myxoedema, the symptoms of which are fatigue, lethargy and increasing sensitivity to cold associated with hoarseness of the voice, swelling of the face and thickening of the skin. The term myxoedema is derived from the nature of the swelling of the skin and subcutaneous tissues which appear to be swollen with a mucin-like product.

Hypothyroidism in the adult may be caused by:

(1) The excision of too great a proportion of thyroid tissue during the operation of subtotal thyroidectomy.
(2) The over-administration of the drugs used in the treatment of hyperthyroidism which block the formation of thyroid hormones. Too large a dose of these drugs leads to iatrogenic myxoedema.
(3) The development of Hashimoto's disease, which causes destruction of the thyroid tissue.

In severe hypothyroidism COMA, HYPOTHERMIA and HEART FAILURE may occur.

Hysteria

A complex psychological disorder in which an individual develops the symptoms and/or signs of loss of bodily function in the absence of organic disease. Two main groups of hysterics are encountered. The individual may develop a derangement of consciousness or memory passing into a trance, STUPOR or FUGUE. Alternatively the hysteric may develop signs of PARALYSIS or the symptoms of a sensory defect. The common paralytic symptoms associated with hysteria include APHONIA (inability to speak). The common sensory defects include blindness, DEAFNESS or an impairment of cutaneous sensation.

Characteristically a hysteric develops symptoms or becomes much worse when in a public place.

Icterus see JAUNDICE

Idiocy

A sign of severe brain damage in which mental retardation to an intelligence quotient of less than 25 occurs.

Idiocy may result from malformations of the brain of unknown cause, from prenatal infections such as rubella, intrauterine ANOXIA and KERNICTERUS. It may also be associated with INBORN ERRORS OF METABOLISM such as phenylketonuria or chromosomal abnormalities such as DOWN'S SYNDROME.

Immunity

Immunity is a sign that the body is able to resist the effects of bacterial or viral infection. Immunity may be innate or acquired. An example of innate immunity is the disease of distemper which affects dogs but not man.

Immunity to an infection usually depends upon the presence in the blood of antibodies to the specific antigens of infecting organisms. Immunity is specific, e.g. a person who has developed antibodies to the typhoid organism is immune to typhoid, but the presence of these particular antibodies does not protect him against other infections.

There are 2 main types of acquired immunity, the distinction depending upon whether the circulating antibodies have been formed by the individual's own body or merely introduced into the circulation:

(1) If the antibodies have been formed following the introduction of antigen into the body a condition of active immunity exists.

(2) If immunity has been produced by injecting antibodies into an individual which have been manufactured either in another individual or more usually an animal, a state

119

of passive immunity exists because no response has been required by the recipient.

Imperforate anus

A sign that a malformation of the cloacal region has occurred in the developing embryo.

When the abnormality is restricted to the anal canal itself, no other malformation may be present, but if the rectum is also involved other abnormalities are commonly present. These include FISTULAE into the vagina in the female or prostatic urethra of the male, incomplete development of the sacrum and pelvic diaphragm and anomalies of the upper urinary tract.

Regardless of the extent of the anomalies, the first danger such a neonate faces is that of intestinal obstruction with its attendant VOMITING.

Inborn errors of metabolism

The term given to a group of diseases all of which are a sign of an inherited failure by the body to synthesize specific enzymes. Such enzyme deficiencies may affect the metabolism of carbohydrates, amino acids or fats and as a result a variety of different diseases are caused, all of which are fortunately rare.

Typical examples of the conditions which may be caused include:

(1) ALKAPTONURIA and PHENYLKETONURIA if amino acid metabolism is affected.
(2) Glycogen storage diseases and GALACTOSAEMIA when carbohydrate metabolism is deranged.
(3) Familial hyper-β-lipoproteinaemia, a condition leading to the early onset of atherosclerosis when fat metabolism is disturbed.

Incontinence of urine

The involuntary passage of urine may be a symptom or sign of many different conditions:

(1) In infancy. Incontinence is normal because the various nervous pathways from the brain to the spinal centres

controlling micturition are not established until comparatively late. However, the great majority of infants are dry both by day and night by the age of four. Regular bed wetting in a 6-year-old can be regarded as abnormal and is known as enuresis. In only about 10 per cent of such infants is there either a well-marked emotional or anatomical reason for the continued incontinence. These may include an emotional reaction to over-strict training or anatomical abnormalities including congenital anomalies of the spinal cord such as a myelomeningocoele which is usually recognized at birth, or a double ureter, one of which opens below the level of the bladder sphincters.

(2) In the adult, incontinence is often classified as true or false. False incontinence is associated with chronic retention so that urine dribbles from the over-distended bladder causing soiling.

True incontinence may be a sign of:

(1) Nervous conditions:

(a) Cerebral. Interference with the conscious level from any cause such as head injury, cerebral HAEMORRHAGE or poisoning may lead to incontinence although this is commonly the result of over-distension due to failure to appreciate the presence of a full bladder. Incontinence is also common in senility associated with cerebral ATROPHY due to loss of central inhibition.

(b) Spinal cord. The spinal cord may be damaged by injuries to the vertebral column. If a complete transection occurs the bladder fills and then overflows during the stage of spinal shock. Following recovery from this stage the precise urinary abnormality depends on the level of the spinal lesion. Complete lack of bladder control follows injuries involving the third, fourth and fifth sacral segments of the cord. Above this level the bladder may become hyperactive responding to smaller than normal quantities of urine. Neurological conditions such as multiple sclerosis may specifically interrupt the inhibitory nerve tracts in the spinal cord.

(2) Laxity of the pelvic diaphragm is a particularly common cause of incontinence in parous women and is due to relaxation of the supporting tissues in the pelvic diaphragm. This leads to the condition known as stress incontinence in which small quantities of urine escape from the bladder particularly if the intra-abdominal pressure is raised by COUGHING, sneezing or bending.

(3) Damage to the bladder sphincters—an uncommon cause of incontinence which is normally seen in males following prostatectomy.

(4) Fistula formation between the bladder and the vagina. Such fistulae may be traumatic or follow the development and/or treatment of cancer of the cervix.

(5) Infection. Particularly in women acute bacterial infections of the bladder may cause such severe irritation and sensitivity of the bladder to distension that the degree of frequency amounts to incontinence.

Chronic infections of the bladder such as uncontrolled tuberculosis may lead to such severe contraction of the bladder that it no longer has any storage capacity. The result is continuous incontinence.

Indigestion see EPIGASTRIC PAIN

Inflammation

A sign of tissue injury caused by bacteria, trauma, chemical agents, viruses, parasites and irradiation. The inflammatory reaction may be acute or chronic.

Acute inflammation is accompanied by pain, swelling, redness and heat in the affected part due to dilatation of the blood vessels and the accumulation in the tissues of an exudate rich in polymorphonuclear leucocytes.

The end result of inflammation depends upon the magnitude of the tissue damage. Minimal inflammation may terminate in complete resolution, the tissues returning to normal. Severe inflammation, however, in which the body's defences are overwhelmed may terminate in ABSCESS formation or SEPTICAEMIA.

Chronic inflammation may follow an acute episode or may be chronic from the outset. Examples of chronic bacterial inflammation include infection with the mycobacteria causing tuberculosis or leprosy. An example of chronic following acute inflammation is improperly or imperfectly treated infection of bone, osteomyelitis. Chronic bacterial inflammation even when involving the skin and subcutaneous tissues is rarely painful although there may be considerable swelling due to the accumulation of lymphocytes in the affected tissues. Damage occurring in the course of chronic inflammation rarely permits a complete return of the tissues to normal even when the infection has been eliminated. The end result of chronic inflammation is one of scarring and fibrosis.

Insomnia

Lack of sleep is a relative condition since the amount required decreases with advancing age.

In adults insomnia may take one of two forms, failure to fall asleep or early waking. Inability to achieve sleep may be caused by environmental factors, by PAIN, worry or excitement. Early waking may also be due to simple environmental causes such as the early morning bird song in summer, but it is a prominent symptom of depression. Physical illness predisposing to early waking includes ulcer dyspepsia, backache, DYSPNOEA or a full bladder due to partial retention caused by prostatism.

Inspiration associated with indrawing of the intercostal spaces

Indrawing of the intercostal spaces during the inspiratory phase of respiration is a sign of severe airway obstruction and is usually much more obvious in children than in adults.

Indrawing is a result of an increase in the negative intrathoracic pressure which is developed in an attempt to overcome the obstruction of the airway.

PARADOXICAL RESPIRATION in which only limited segments of the chest wall or sternum move inwards instead of outwards on inspiration occurs following severe injuries to the chest.

Intersex

A condition in which the sex of a neonate is in doubt at the time of birth. A female intersex usually follows congenital adrenal hyperplasia or more rarely the administration of androgenic hormones to a mother during early pregnancy. The clitoris is enlarged and the labia may be fused together, thus obscuring the vaginal orifice. A male intersex occurs if the testicles have failed to secrete sufficient androgenic hormones to develop the masculine external genitalia. The correct sex of such an infant can be established by studies of the chromosomes and biopsy of the gonads.

Intracranial pressure, increase in

The pressure within the cranial cavity is usually indirectly estimated by measuring the pressure of the cerebrospinal fluid in the subarachnoid space by a lumbar puncture. This pressure is normally below 150 mm of water.

A lumbar puncture, for this purpose, is performed with the patient lying on the side. The needle is inserted into the subarachnoid space between the spinous processes of the second and third or the third and fourth lumbar vertebrae. Once the stillette is removed fluid should freely drip from the needle after which a simple glass manometer is attached.

The patency of the subarachnoid space through which the cerebrospinal fluid circulates is gauged by Queckenstedt's test in which the internal jugular veins in the neck are occluded by compression. In a normal individual the recorded pressure in the manometer then rises because of the rise in pressure in the intracranial veins and capillaries.

If examination of a patient has already demonstrated the presence of PAPILLOEDEMA, which is commonly caused by a raised intracranial pressure, great care must be taken when performing a lumbar puncture since coning may occur.

The common causes of a raised intracranial pressure are:

(1) Space-occupying lesions such as intracranial tumours affecting the meninges or the brain.

(2) Bleeding into the extradural, subdural or subarachnoid spaces or even into the brain itself caused by rupture of

an atherosclerotic or aneurysmal cerebral artery or by injury.
(3) OEDEMA of the brain following severe injury.
(4) Congenital malformations preventing the normal circulation of cerebrospinal fluid and thus causing hydrocephalus.

The symptoms produced by a raised intracranial pressure include:
(1) HEADACHE, usually occurring in paroxysms of great severity often with periods of freedom.
(2) VOMITING which is typically not preceded by NAUSEA and which may be projectile in type.
(3) Mental confusion finally terminating in COMA.

The signs depend upon the nature of the causative lesion, but in all patients the following are common:
(1) Papilloedema leading to a variety of visual defects.
(2) BRADYCARDIA.
(3) Respiratory arrhythmia passing to CHEYNE-STOKES RESPIRATIONS.
(4) Generalized CONVULSIONS.

Unrelieved raised intracranial pressure may eventually cause coma and finally death. In hydrocephalus, the increased pressure within the ventricles of the brain cause their gradual distension, with the result that the head enlarges and the actual brain tissue atrophies leading to mental retardation should the child survive.

Jaundice

A symptom of disease caused by the retention of bile pigments in the blood so that a yellow or greenish yellow discoloration of the skin, sclera and tissues generally occurs. The level of bilirubin in the serum of a normal individual is 0.5 to 1.0 mg per cent (8–16 μmol/litre); a concentration above 2 mg per cent results in obvious jaundice.

There are 3 basic causes of jaundice;
(1) Excessive breakdown of erythrocytes (haemolysis) from any cause leads to an increased concentration of bile

pigment in the plasma. This is pre-hepatic jaundice. Causes of haemolytic jaundice include: congenital spherocytosis in which the erythrocytes are abnormal and more easily haemolysed than the normal; incompatible blood transfusion in which the incompatible donor cells are destroyed by antibodies in the recipient's blood.

(2) Damage to the liver itself. This leads to the liver cells being unable to excrete bile pigment brought to them in the circulation. This type is commonly called hepatic or liver cell jaundice. A common cause of hepatic jaundice is viral hepatitis, but it may also follow the accidental or deliberate administration of chemical substances which poison and therefore damage the liver cells, such as carbon tetrachloride, halothane or alcohol. The latter may cause such severe damage to the liver, when taken in excess over a long period, that cirrhosis develops.

(3) The outflow of bile from the liver is obstructed. The outflow block may be within the liver itself involving the bile canaliculi or it may originate in the extra-hepatic biliary system, i.e. the common hepatic ducts or common bile duct. This type of jaundice is known as obstructive jaundice and common causes of this type of jaundice include stones in the common bile duct and cancer in the head of the pancreas.

Jaundice may be associated with symptoms and signs which suggest in which of the above categories it belongs. The following symptoms and signs occur in obstructive jaundice:

(1) ABDOMINAL PAIN, BILIARY COLIC.

(2) STEATORRHOEA due to the absence of bile salts from the gastrointestinal tract.

(3) Excessive bleeding due to a vitamin K deficiency.

(4) Discoloration of the urine due to the presence of bile pigment.

(5) The gall bladder may be palpable if the point of obstruction is below the level of junction of the cystic duct with the common hepatic duct, i.e. lies in the common bile duct.

See also ACHOLURIC JAUNDICE.

Jugular vein engorgement

Normally veins above the level of the junction of the manubrium with the body of the sternum whether sitting or standing are collapsed whereas veins below this level are filled.

When an individual is supine with the head on 2 or 3 pillows, the level of blood reaches about one-third of the way up the neck, a level which will be found to correspond with the level of the sternal angle.

In patients suffering from congestive HEART FAILURE, in which the right ventricle fails to function, the consequent obstruction to the return of blood to the heart leads to distension of the jugular vein so that even when standing a column of blood may still be visible and pulsatile.

Other less common causes of jugular vein engorgement include:

(1) Obstruction of the superior vena cava by tumours of the superior mediastinum. Such engorgement is not pulsatile and is due to the tumour interfering with the flow of blood from the jugular veins to the right atrium.

(2) Constrictive pericarditis in which the gradual contraction of the pericardial sac slowly hinders the free return of blood to the right atrium.

Kernicterus

A form of severe JAUNDICE in the newborn, usually a sign of severe and excessive haemolysis of the infant's erythrocytes. The haemolysing agent is the antibody to the Rhesus factor and the excessive bilirubin in the circulation not only leads to jaundice but also to brain damage from the effect of the bile pigments on the brain.

Should the infant survive some degree of mental retardation usually follows. It is interesting that this type of neonatal brain damage does not occur in babies suffering from obstructive jaundice due to atresia of the bile ducts. This is because in the latter condition the excess bile pigments have passed through the liver cells and their chemical composition has been so changed that they can no longer pass across the blood–brain barrier and affect the brain cells.

The Rhesus factor is a blood-group antigen present in the red blood cells of 85 per cent of the population. If a Rhesus-negative female becomes pregnant and her baby is Rhesus positive, the mother will be stimulated to form anti-Rhesus antibodies. These are not normally present in sufficient quantities to affect the first pregnancy, but should she become pregnant again and the second fetus is also Rhesus positive more antibodies are formed and some begin to pass through the placenta to cause haemolysis of the baby's erythrocytes. This is the underlying cause of the condition of erythroblastosis fetalis. Kernicterus implies that bile pigment has been deposited in the brain.

Kernig's sign

A sign indicating the presence of irritation or INFLAMMATION of the meninges, the common causes of which are either meningitis or subarachnoid HAEMORRHAGE.

In the presence of either, full extension of the knee is impossible when the hip is flexed to about 90° due to spasm of the hamstring muscles at the back of the thigh.

Ketonuria

The presence of ketone bodies in the urine is a sign of ketosis which is a frequent complication of diabetes mellitus. This is due to the inefficient metabolism of fatty acids because of absence or relative lack of the hormone insulin.

The presence of ketone bodies in the urine can be established by the use of various chemical reagents.

Ketosis

A sign commonly seen in untreated or inadequately treated diabetes mellitus in which ketone bodies such as acetone and aceto-acetic acid accumulate in the blood stream due to the inefficient metabolism of fat.

The onset of ketosis is associated with malaise, rapid breathing, anorexia, and thirst, followed later by VOMITING, DEHYDRATION, air hunger, abdominal pain and finally COMA. All these symptoms occur because of the severe metabolic ACIDOSIS which accompanies this condition. Ketosis can often be recognized by the smell of ketone bodies on the breath, likened to the smell of peardrops.

Kleinfelter's syndrome

A syndrome due to a chromosomal abnormality in which there is additional X or sex chromosome material present in the cells.

Many examples of this syndrome first come to light when an affected male complains of infertility. An increase in X chromosomes in the male produces a tendency to mental subnormality. The external genitalia are usually normal in appearance despite testicular ATROPHY and some GYNAECOMASTIA.

Koilonychia

A sign indicating the presence of an iron-deficiency ANAEMIA in which the fingernails are brittle, have a tendency to split and possess a flatness or even a concavity.

Any cause of iron deficiency may be associated with this type of nail deformity and, when the anaemia is severe, stomatitis and glossitis may also occur, leading to soreness of the mouth and difficulty in chewing.

Korsakoff's syndrome

A syndrome observed in chronic alcoholics due to the absence of the enzyme thiamine. The patient develops a loss of memory for extremely recent events which cannot be readily recalled with the result that intelligent planning becomes impossible. This is because thoughts or ideas rapidly disappear from the intellect as a plan of action takes shape. A similar condition is occasionally seen in other intoxications and infections.

Kyphosis

A curvature of the spine in an antero-posterior axis. The curvature may be smooth or angular, mobile or fixed.

A kyphos may be a sign of:

(1) Poor posture, which gives rise to a smooth mobile kyphosis which can be corrected by lying down or by a conscious effort to stand erect.
(2) Previous poliomyelitis, because this infection may cause

paralysis of those muscles of the spine concerned with maintaining the erect position.

(3) Scheuermann's disease, or adolescent kyphosis in which the epiphyses of the vertebral bodies become partially separated from the underlying bone.

(4) Ankylosing spondylitis, a disease of unknown cause in which a progressive inflammatory disease affecting the joints of the spine occurs, leading to a slowly increasing kyphosis. Untreated this condition leads to a character-istic 'hangdog' appearance.

(5) Osteoporosis, a condition of bone in which the quality and basic architecture remain but the amount becomes smaller. The commonest cause of osteoporosis is the hormonal imbalance which follows the menopause, a condition known as post-menopausal osteoporosis. Osteoporosis, however, may accompany or complicate a variety of disease conditions including CUSHING'S SYN-DROME, chronic liver disease or the over-enthusiastic use of corticosteroid hormones. The development of post-menopausal osteoporosis accounts for the frequency of fracture of the neck of the femur in the ageing female.

(6) Infections of the spinal column. Tuberculosis of the spine, now rare in Europe, is the commonest cause of an angu-lar kyphos. This infection commonly attacks the thoraco-lumbar region of the spine causing destruction of the vertebral bodies. The actual point of angulation is known as the gibbus.

(7) Injuries to the spine.

(8) The commonest cause of an angular kyphos in highly developed countries is the presence of metastatic malig-nant disease affecting the spine, the most frequent site of the primary being the breast.

Leukoplakia

White thickened patches of mucous membranes involving the buccal mucosa, tongue, penis or vulva. In some individuals it is a sign of a late syphilitic infection. In the mouth and on the lips leukoplakia is seen most commonly in elderly pipe smokers due to the action of the tars in the tobacco which stimulate a reaction in the epithelium, with which they come in contact. The result in such patients is the subsequent development of cancer in the affected areas. The onset of malignancy can often be detected by the naked eye when inspection reveals that the white patches are becoming FISSURED.

Lid lag

Otherwise known as von Graefe's sign lid lag is present only in thyrotoxicosis. The sign is elicited by fixing the head of the affected individual and then asking him to watch a finger moving first upwards and then downwards. As the eyes follow the finger downwards, so the upper eyelids lag behind leaving the sclera visible above the iris. This sign is caused by the excessive circulating thyroid hormone stimulating the sympathetic nervous system which supplies fibres to the levator palpebrae superioris which, in part, controls movements of the upper eyelid.

This sign may be present even in the absence of true EXOPH-THALMOS.

Lower motor neurone, signs of disease

The lower motor neurones originate from cell bodies situated in the anterior (ventral) horn of the grey matter of the spinal cord.

Signs that such neurones have been damaged by disease or injury include:

(1) PARALYSIS and flaccidity of individual muscles or groups of muscles.
(2) Profound wasting of the affected muscles which have been deprived of their nerve supply.
(3) Diminished or absent tendon reflexes.
(4) Lack of associated muscle tone in the muscles affected.
(5) Trophic changes due mainly to the associated damage to the sensory and autonomic fibres which are carried with the motor nerve fibres in the peripheral nerves. The major trophic changes include a cold blue shiny skin sometimes accompanied by ULCERATION.

A once common cause of lower motor neurone disease was

the virus responsible for poliomyelitis which has an affinity for the cells from which the motor nerve fibres take origin in the spinal cord. Since the introduction of vaccines and the routine immunization of all children, the paralytic form of this disease has become uncommon.

Lymphoedema

A form of swelling caused by the accumulation of lymph in the skin and subcutaneous tissues. Unlike OEDEMA, lymphoedema does not pit on pressure.

It may be a sign of a congenital absence of the lymphatic vessels, in the leg causing Milroy's disease. It may be the result of blockage of the lymphatics, commonly by malignant deposits in the lymph nodes, or rarely by parasites such as the nematode worm. This worm causes the clinical condition known as filariasis. The affected lymph nodes in which the worm ledges are enlarged and the tissues distal to them are grossly swollen by lymphoedema.

Macroglossia

Enlargement of the tongue which may be painless or painful. Painless enlargement of congenital origin occurs in cretins, congenital HYPOTHYROIDISM, and DOWN'S SYNDROME. Acquired enlargement occurs in acromegaly.

Painful enlargement may occur in the course of an acute oropharyngeal infection or as the result of nutritional deficiency (a dietary lack of iron, folic acid, nicotinic acid and riboflavine may lead to a painful, enlarged, fissured tongue).

Mallory-Weiss syndrome

Severe upper gastrointestinal bleeding originating from mucosal tears of the lower end of the oesophagus. These are usually the result of severe VOMITING and so any situation in which vomiting is commonplace or severe may precipitate this type of HAEMORRHAGE. Examples include acute alcoholic poisoning, peptic ulceration and hiatus hernia. The oesophagus need not necessarily be diseased.

Mania

An affective disorder of the mind in which the mood of elation is more than that of a comfortable sense of well-being. The characteristic feature of the manic mood is its extreme variability, at one moment the patient may appear to be normally elated and at the next the patient has become aggressively angry with a total loss of social inhibitions.

Thinking is accelerated and fragmented, thoughts translated into speech are uttered with no pause for reflection upon their effect on the recipient. The result of the ill-considered thought is errors in reasoning and judgement. Underlining this apparently intense mental activity is an inability to sustain concentration, reading is abandoned, but writing letters full of exclamation marks and dogmatic over-statements may occur.

Mania is more serious than depression but complete recovery normally occurs, particularly in young persons.

There is some evidence that mania may be the result of changes in the way in which the brain metabolizes or releases those chemical compounds which transmit impulses between the various neurones, particularly of the autonomic nervous system, the compounds which are collectively known as the biogenic amines.

Marasmus

A sign of extreme starvation in childhood when the diet is grossly deficient in energy-giving foods and also fails to meet the protein requirements. The marasmic infant fails to thrive, is irritable or apathetic and may suffer from both DIARRHOEA and VOMITING.

The child is shrunken and wizened due to the complete absence of subcutaneous fat. The muscles are atrophic and therefore weak.

Meig's syndrome

An uncommon syndrome in which a pleural effusion together with ASCITES occurs in association with a benign ovarian tumour known as a fibroma.

Melaena

A dark, tarry, loose stool due to the presence of altered blood from a haemorrhage arising from the upper part of the gastrointestinal tract, including the upper jejunum.

The common causes giving rise to melaena include:

(1) Chronic peptic ULCERATION of the stomach or duodenum which accounts for approximately half of all cases.

(2) Acute erosion of the stomach from an unknown cause or precipitated by drugs such as butazolidine or aspirin.

(3) Oesophageal varices.

The actual character of the stool depends on the site of bleeding, the amount of blood and the time taken for the blood to pass through the gastrointestinal tract. If the bleeding is severe and occurs above the duodenal-jejunal flexure, HAEMATEMESIS results. Melaena, when severe, gives rise to DIARRHOEA and may cause hypovolaemic SHOCK.

Mendelson's syndrome

A combination of respiratory failure and SHOCK following the aspiration of gastric contents into the respiratory passage, usually during the induction of anaesthesia in obstetrical patients or patients suffering severe intestinal obstruction. The highly acid gastric contents provoke a severe INFLAMMATION of the bronchial tree, thus leading to respiratory complications.

Meningismus

The term given to a condition in which the signs of meningeal irritation are present without any actual INFLAMMATION of the meninges. The positive signs found include neck rigidity and a positive KERNIG'S sign.

Meningismus is common in pneumonia, particularly in young children.

Menorrhagia

Abnormal uterine HAEMORRHAGE occurring at the normal cyclical period but being excessive in both amount and duration.

This type of bleeding is usually caused by conditions in which the area of endometrium, that is the surface available for bleeding, is increased by conditions such as uterine fibroids or the condition of adenomyosis. It may also be a symptom of a blood disease characterized by faulty clotting such as aplastic ANAEMIA, leukaemia, thrombocytopenic PURPURA or HAEMOPHILIA.

Moon-face

The term given to the fat rounded face associated with CUSHING'S SYNDROME, but also more frequently caused by the over-administration of glucocorticoids. The affected individual also exhibits the specific OBESITY seen in these conditions occurring only on the trunk and proximal portions of the limbs.

Munchausen's syndrome

The patient who wanders from hospital to hospital with the symptoms and even the signs of physical abdominal disease. Several bear numerous scars, testimony to the convincing manner in which they tell their respective stories. Commonly the individual gives a different name in the different hospitals he or she attends, making tracing difficult. One of the authors had a woman who had succeeded in being admitted to several hospitals both abroad and at home. She bore 7 abdominal scars and convinced the author she required another laparotomy and then refused surgery.

Murphy's sign

A sign present in patients suffering from acute INFLAMMATION of the gall bladder. The examiner presses his fingers gently but firmly over the right subcostal region and asks the patient to take a slow deep breath. As the inflamed gall bladder strikes the peritoneum beneath the examining fingers a momentary interruption of breathing occurs because of the increased PAIN. This sign should be combined with Boas' sign which consists of hyperaesthesia of the skin to pin prick over the tip of the right scapula.

135

Muscular atrophy

Muscular atrophy may occur in the absence of nervous disease. This is a sign of a group of diseases known as the muscular dystrophies, all of which are of a familial nature and all of which usually make their appearance in childhood or early adolescence. In many patients, although the power of the muscles diminishes, there may be apparent hypertrophy, known as pseudohypertrophy, because the increase in size is not due to an increase or enlargement of muscle fibres in the muscle, but to an overgrowth of fat and connective tissue.

Conditions illustrating these features occur in:

Pseudohypertrophic muscular dystrophy. The muscular weakness first affects the pelvic girdle and is manifest within the first 3 years of life. Pseudohypertrophy of the calves and deltoid appears. By the age of 10 most of the affected children, who are mostly boys, are unable to walk and the majority die within 20 years.

Facio-scapulo humeral muscular dystrophy. A benign condition presenting usually between 10 and 20 years of age, often with weakness of the facial muscles followed by similar loss of strength in the muscles of the shoulder girdle. There may be little functional weakness, but the involvement of the face gives rise to an unattractive appearance particularly when smiling.

Nausea

A desire to vomit without actually VOMITING in which a feeling of unease is felt in the abdomen, often associated with sweating, excessive salivation and extreme malaise. In many patients nausea is followed by vomiting, the latter act eventually relieving the unpleasant sensation of nausea.

Conditions in which nausea occurs which are not necessarily followed by vomiting include benign and malignant ULCERATION of the stomach, benign ulceration of the duodenum, pregnancy and diseases affecting the labyrinthine system of the inner ear. Commoner perhaps than all these organic conditions is dietary over-indulgence, usually through the excessive intake of alcohol.

Neck rigidity

A sign indicating irritation or INFLAMMATION of the meninges (see KERNIG'S SIGN). Neck rigidity is caused by spasm of the extensor muscles of the neck and spine. In severe cases the head is even retracted and in severer cases still the back may be arched creating the condition of OPISTHOTONOS.

Neck rigidity is also present in fractures of the cervical spine in which, unassociated with any other injury, the patient may sit holding his head in his hands.

Neuropathic joint

The painless grossly disorganized joint seen in a variety of neurological conditions in all of which pain and proprioceptive sensation is lost from the joint and its capsule.

Characteristically the following diseases and joints are involved: diabetic neuropathy affecting the ankle joint, tabes dorsalis, the knee and hip joints, and syringomyelia, the shoulder and elbow. The derangement arises because, in the absence of sensation, no reflex safeguard against injury can occur.

The symptoms associated with a neuropathic joint include weakness due to ATROPHY of the surrounding muscles, instability because of damage to the surrounding ligaments, swelling due to effusion and excess bone formation and deformity due to a combination of these factors.

Nocturia

The disturbance of an individual's sleep by the need to micturate.

The symptom is most commonly caused by conditions which lead to increasing sensitivity of the bladder wall to distension, as in cystitis; it may also occur because the bladder wall is being persistently irritated by a vesical calculus or because the size of the bladder has been so reduced that it is unable to hold any adequate quantity of urine. This is usually the end result of chronic infections such as tuberculosis or schistosomiasis which can cause severe fibrosis of the vesical wall.

137

In males prostatic hypertrophy is a common cause of nocturia, either because secondary infection has occurred or because the improper emptying of the bladder causes a gradual reduction in the functional storage capacity of the bladder. Thus if the residual urine after micturition in 100 ml and the normal bladder capacity is only 300 ml, micturition will be initiated when only 200 ml of urine have been added to the residual.

Nodules, Heberden's see HERBERDEN'S NODULES

Nystagmus

An uncontrollable oscillation of the eyeball usually in a lateral but occasionally in a rotary direction.

Nystagmus may be a sign of a disturbance of visual function, of labyrinthine function or of the central nervous system. The oscillatory movements may be regular with an equal arc of movement to either side at exactly the same speed, or they may be jerky with a rapid movement to one side and a slow movement back to the opposite side.

Nystagmus sometimes occurs in the absence of any organic lesion, the best known example being railway nystagmus, known as optokinetic nystagmus, which appears when a passenger looks out through the train window at the passing scenery. His eyes slowly follow objects which are passing and when these reach the limit of his vision his eyes quickly flash back to the opposite extreme and the movement begins again. In congenital blindness since the eyes lack a focal point they oscillate aimlessly. In labyrinthine disturbances, since there are 3 semicircular canals it is possible for nystagmus to be in any one of 3 directions depending on the particular canal or canals affected.

When the disturbance causing the nystagmus lies in the brain, the movements are usually finer and of a less regular nature. Any condition affecting vestibular connections between the brain stem and cerebellum may result in nystagmus. This ocular disturbance is therefore common in syringobulbia, tumours of this area of the brain, multiple sclerosis and degenerative lesions caused by atherosclerosis of the vertebral or basilar arteries.

Obesity

Obesity defined as an excess of fat in the body only occurs when the intake of energy-giving foods exceeds the energy utilized by the work of the body and the energy output by physical activity. Obesity is a common accompaniment of middle age but in some families it may occur much earlier, probably due to a combination of hereditary and social factors.

Obesity, not itself caused by disease, is of great importance in the development of a variety of conditions including diabetes, atheroma of the arterial system and hiatus hernia. Furthermore, the presence of obesity increases the work of the heart and therefore aggravates DYSPNOEA, whatever its cause.

The development of obesity in a previously healthy individual may be a sign of:

(1) Psychological disturbance. Both stress or depressive situations may lead the affected individual to eat excessively with the result that a rapid weight gain occurs. Note the rapid development of obesity which occurs in normal individuals who cease smoking.

(2) Endocrine disturbances.
   (a) Adrenal. CUSHING'S SYNDROME or disease is associated with a proximal accretion of fat in the trunk and limbs.
   (b) Pituitary—hypothalamic disturbances are associated with obesity, see FROHLICH'S SYNDROME.
   (c) Eunuchoidism, loss of male hormone leads to increasing obesity in the affected male.

(3) Rare disturbances known as the lipodystrophies in which particular parts of the body may be affected. In the commonest type of this rare condition the fat from the upper half of the body tends to waste whilst the lower limbs tend, paradoxically, to be fatter than usual.

(4) Dercum's disease, which usually occurs in obese menopausal women and is a condition characterized by the development of multiple painful indurated plaques in the subcutaneous fat.

When the obesity is generalized, its degree can be calculated either by comparing the known weight of the individual against standard charts, or by measuring the skinfold thickness, usually over the biceps muscle of the arm.

Obsession, obsessional personality

Obsessions are ideas, images or urges which are accompanied by a feeling of domination, strongly resisted and recognized by a person as irrational. Obsessions may occur alone but are more commonly associated with a variety of psychiatric disorders such as schizophrenia and depression.

An obsession can be so disturbing that it interferes with normal living. An obsession is often associated with fears (phobias) one of the better known of which is fear of uncleanliness which gives rise to repeated washing without cause. Such an act may be accompanied by a compulsive ritual, e.g. the order in which the washing is carried out must always be adhered to and if deviated from, a start must be made again from the beginning.

Obsessional behaviour occurs in quite normal people who may exhibit a number of well-recognized traits such as orderliness, frugality and obstinacy. Such individuals are often beset by a feeling of insecurity which leads to desire for total perfection, hence the term, perfectionist. Unfortunately this admirable trait is often nullified by their obstinacy and rigidity of mind.

Oedema

Oedema is defined as the excessive extravascular accumulation of fluid although in its usual context the term is applied only to fluid accumulating in the interstitial tissues. Fluid accumulating in the various cavities of the body such as the ventricles of the brain, the pleural or peritoneal cavities is referred to under specific titles, hydrocephalus, pleural effusion or ASCITES.

The subcutaneous tissues affected by oedema may or may not pit on pressure. This sign is elicited by attempting to indent the affected area by finger pressure. If on removal of the finger a surface indentation remains the oedema is referred to as pitting. A non-pitting oedema is evidence of long-standing oedema or of LYMPHOEDEMA. Oedema may be local or general. Common causes of local oedema include:

(1) Acute INFLAMMATION. Inflammatory oedema is produced by the leakage of protein molecules from the capillaries damaged by the inflammatory process. This increases the osmotic pressure in the tissues outside the capillaries and fluid is drawn from the vessels into the tissues.

(2) ALLERGY, URTICARIA is an example of allergic oedema.

(3) Obstruction to the venous drainage of a particular area. This type of oedema is caused by the rising venous pressure causing an increase in capillary pressure of such a degree that fluid is forced out from the capillaries. Such oedema is seen in individuals suffering from valvular incompetence of the veins of the lower limb.

(4) Lymphoedema.

The common causes of more generalized oedema include:

(1) CARDIAC FAILURE.

(2) Hypoproteinaemia. Any condition causing a reduction in the amount of protein in the circulation leads to oedema due to the reduction of the osmotic pressure within the capillaries. Hypoproteinaemia may follow:

(a) Starvation leading to famine oedema.

(b) Kwashiorkor, a condition affecting infants in certain parts of the world after weaning caused by feeding the infants on dilute cereal gruels low in protein. In contrast to marasmus, which is the childhood equivalent to adult starvation, the diet may provide an adequate or nearly adequate amount of energy.

(c) Inflammatory diseases of the bowel such as occur in the ZOLLINGER–ELLISON SYNDROME may lead to profound losses of protein from the mucosa of the gut. Collectively these conditions are known as the protein-losing enteropathies.

(d) Renal oedema. In acute glomerular nephritis for reasons as yet unknown sodium is retained in the body and with it water leading to generalized oedema. In the nephrotic syndrome which may

141

follow acute nephritis the situation is made worse by the loss of protein which occurs from the kidneys and the secretion of the hormone known as aldosterone which increases sodium retention in the body.

See also ANGIO-NEUROTIC OEDEMA.

Oligaemia

A reduction in the circulating blood volume, which is normally approximately 5 litres in an adult.

Oligaemia is produced by any condition which causes a sudden loss of fluid from the body.

(1) Haemorrhage.
(2) Loss of plasma following a severe burn.
(3) Loss of fluid and electrolytes due to VOMITING in a patient suffering from an intestinal obstruction.

Severe oligaemia is alway followed by SHOCK, oliguria and commonly by ANAEMIA if the cause is bleeding.

Opisthotonos

A sign of intense spasm of the extensor muscles of the neck and back which when severe may cause the back to become so arched that an affected person may rest on his head and his heels.

The commonest cause of opisthotonos is TETANUS, a disease caused by infection with the bacterium, *Clostridium tetani*. This organism once it has invaded the tissues and is in a suitable anaerobic environment, produces an exotoxin known as tetanospasmin. This travels along the motor nerves in the vicinity and causes spasm of the muscles supplied by them, in this case the muscles of the back. A similar condition may be caused by strychnine poisoning although the precise mode of action of this drug is unknown.

Optic atrophy

Optic atrophy is a sign of a variety of conditions affecting the eye and the optic nerve. These include retinal disease, injury to the optic nerve, diseases affecting the optic nerve including

142

multiple sclerosis, unrelieved PAPILLOEDEMA and thrombosis of the central artery of the retina.

Optic atrophy is accompanied by severe visual impairment or even blindness and examination of the retina by means of an ophthalmoscope reveals that the optic disc is paler than normal. Its margins may be well defined or blurred, depending on the underlying cause.

Orthopnoea

Orthopnoea describes a breathlessness developing when lying flat in bed which is relieved by sleeping in the sitting position. This symptom only occurs in HEART FAILURE and is usually associated with paroxysmal nocturnal DYSPNOEA or CARDIAC ASTHMA.

The symptom arises because there is a shift of blood in the recumbent position from the splanchnic area and legs to the upper half of the body. This leads to an increase in pulmonary congestion, a decrease in the elasticity of the lungs and a reduced vital capacity; all factors which increase the effort required to breath.

Otorrhoea, cerebrospinal see CEREBROSPINAL OTORRHOEA

Pain

Pain is a common symptom of disease. Regardless of its cause, the nerve impulses required to excite a painful sensation reach the brain by passing along the fibres in the spinal cord known as the spinothalamic tract to the thalamus. From this area there are widespread connections to other parts of the brain although no precise area has been definitely localized which can be properly named the pain centre.

The structure of the actual nerve endings from which the sensation of pain arises varies considerably; in the skin these are often free whereas in the intestine where the nerve endings chiefly respond to stretch, the nerve endings are complex structures.

When attempting to analyse the cause of a particular pain, attention must be paid to its site, radiation, its time relationships, character, severity, aggravating factors, relieving fac-

tors, associated symptoms and lastly the psychological character of the individual. A few individuals are incapable of feeling
pain regardless of the intensity of the stimulus. In many
patients a careful clinical history will reveal the cause of the
pain, for example the pain patterns occurring in association
with BILIARY COLIC, renal colic or duodenal ulceration are
classical. The nature of the associated symptoms is also of great
importance. For example the presence of fortification spectra
in association with HEADACHE strongly suggests a diagnosis of
migraine.

See also ABDOMINAL PAIN, EPIGASTRIC PAIN, HUNGER PAIN,
REFERRED PAIN, RETROSTERNAL PAIN, SHOULDER-TIP PAIN.

Palpitation

Consciousness of the action of the heart which normally is un-
noticed. The rapid forceful beat of the heart following severe
physical exertion can always be appreciated even in the heal-
thiest individual, and an anxious individual may be conscious
of the heart's action at rest. In normal individuals the commonest cause of palpitations is a sudden change in rate or
rhythm such as occurs with the abrupt onset of TACHYCARDIA
or ATRIAL FIBRILLATION.

Papilloedema

A sign associated with the following conditions:

(1) Raised intracranial pressure.
(2) Tumours of the orbit large enough to compress the
    central vein of the retina.
(3) Thrombosis of the central retinal vein.
(4) HYPERTENSION.

The condition is primarily due to local OEDEMA of the optic
discs, the point on the retina at which the nerve fibres concerned with sight come together to form the optic nerve and
leave the eye, a point at which the retinal artery also reaches
the eye and the retinal vein leaves it.

If the condition is severe the patient complains of blurred
vision and special examination will lead to discovery of enlargement of the blind spot and contraction of the peripheral
part of the visual fields.

Paradoxical respiration

Respiratory movements associated with a portion of the chest wall moving inwards on inspiration and outwards on expiration; the opposite, therefore, of the normal respiratory excursion.

Paradox is a sign of severe injury to the chest wall accompanied by either complete detachment of a number of ribs at both their anterior and posterior extremities, i.e. near the sternum and near the thoracic vertebrae, or alternatively, detachment of the sternum from the rib cage by a series of fractures which usually involve the costochondral junctions on both sides of this bone.

Paradox develops because inspiration is accompanied by a decrease in the intrathoracic pressure which, therefore, sucks the affected part of the chest wall inwards during this respiratory phase.

The severity of the paradox is related to:

(1) The number of ribs detached from the thoracic cage.
(2) The degree of respiratory effort. As this becomes greater so the paradoxical movement becomes more marked.

The presence of paradox is of great importance because the lung tissue underlying the lesion is not aerated even though blood may continue to flow through the underlying lung if this has not been too severely contused. As a result hypoxia followed by DYSPNOEA develops and respiratory failure may eventually lead to coma and death.

The paradoxical movement is usually treated by tracheal intubation and intermittent positive pressure ventilation.

Paraesthesia

Subjective sensations of tingling, 'pins and needles', numbness or burning.

Paraesthesiae are common in FUNCTIONAL disorders and also occur in organic nervous diseases such as multiple sclerosis, sub-acute combined degeneration of the cord, polyneuritis and when a sensory nerve is subjected to pressure. Examples of paraesthesiae following pressure are the tingling in the hand felt in the presence of a cervical rib and the carpal tunnel syndrome. When the distribution of the paraesthesiae corresponds to that of known nerves such as the median nerve, or to a specific segment of the spinal cord, it suggests that the cause of the disordered sensation is organic rather than FUNCTIONAL.

Paralysis

An inability of a muscle or group of muscles to contract.

Paralysis is usually the result of damage to the motor neurones although it can occur if there is interference at the neuromuscular junction. For each muscle to contract at least two motor nerves are involved:

(1) The upper motor neurone which commences with the nerve cell in the motor cortex, travels down the spinal cord in the pyramidal or corticospinal tracts and ends in the anterior (ventral) horn of the spinal cord.

(2) The lower motor neurone, the cell body of which lies in the anterior (ventral) horn of the spinal cord and whose axon passes out to end in the muscle at the motor end plate.

Paralysis may follow damage of either upper or lower motor neurones. Paralysis due to upper motor neurone damage, for example by a STROKE, produces:

(1) A spastic paralysis in which the muscles are more rigid than normal.

(2) Exaggerated reflex actions.

(3) No wasting of the affected muscles.

Paralysis due to a lower motor lesion produces:

(1) A flaccid paralysis in which there is no tone in the muscle, which is 'floppy'.

(2) Absent reflex actions due to the interference with the spinal reflex arc.

(3) Marked muscle wasting.

Conditions causing this type of paralysis include poliomyelitis and spinal injuries.

Sometimes the term PARESIS is confused with paralysis. Paresis indicates that there is a reduction in the power of contraction—weakness in the muscle without total loss of power.

Both paralysis and paresis can occur if there is a fault at the neuromuscular junction, as in the disease of myasthenia gravis.

Paralytic ileus

A sign of paralysis of the smooth muscle of the bowel wall resulting in an interference with the forward flow of the gastrointestinal contents. The common causes of ileus include:

(1) General PERITONITIS, either chemical, e.g. following perforation of a duodenal ulcer, or bacterial, e.g. following appendicitis or diverticulitis.
(2) Severe injuries to the spine causing retroperitoneal haematoma in the region of the sympathetic nerve trunk.
(3) Injuries to the vertebral column associated with spinal cord injury and spinal shock.
(4) Ileus may also sometimes complicate the application of a plaster cast which encloses the whole abdomen, as may be used for the treatment of a prolapsed intervertebral disc.

The underlying causes of ileus, therefore, are principally:

(1) Conditions in which a direct toxic effect is exerted on the gastrointestinal muscle.
(2) Interference with the autonomic nerve supply of the intestinal tract.

The signs of ileus are:

(1) A 'silent' abdomen, listening to the abdomen with a stethoscope reveals no bowel sounds.
(2) Gross abdominal distension.
(3) Severe intractable VOMITING.
(4) Failure to pass either faeces or flatus, the condition of absolute constipation.

Untreated, the patient suffering from ileus may die from the primary cause, for example an untreated peritonitis or from DEHYDRATION.

The term ileus is also used to describe two very rare forms of mechanical obstruction to the bowel.

(1) Duodenal ileus; obstruction of the horizontal part of the duodenum by the superior mesenteric artery which

crosses in front of the horizontal part of the duodenum in its passage to the small bowel mesentery. This type of obstruction usually occurs in thin old women following abdominal surgery.

(2) Gall stone ileus; obstruction to the distal ileum by a large gall stone. The gall stone enters the bowel via a FISTULA between the gall bladder and the duodenum which usually follows a severe attack of cholecystitis.

Paranoia

A mental disorder in which the affected individual slowly develops a DELUSION although retaining perfectly orderly thinking. Should the delusion relate to treachery or injustice such a person may become extremely dangerous as he or she seeks revenge. Another common delusion is a morbid jealousy, particularly of a spouse. Seen more commonly in men than in women this symptom often begins in early middle life.

A paranoid reaction, i.e. a suspicion of environmental hostility or criticism may occur in any systemic illness, especially those associated with alterations in cerebral metabolism, e.g. hypoxia due to cardiac or respiratory failure or any metabolic disturbance leading to ACIDOSIS. In the elderly, paranoia is commonplace in cerebral ATROPHY following cerebral atherosclerosis.

Paraplegia

A sign of spinal cord damage leading to a PARALYSIS of both lower limbs. The paralysis may develop rapidly following an injury to the spinal cord or sudden arrest of the circulation to the cord, or more slowly as in disseminated sclerosis in which increasing numbers of nerve fibres cease to function and later degenerate due to the loss of their myelin sheaths.

Paresis

A term implying weakness rather than paralysis of a single muscle or group of muscles concerned with a particular movement.

The presence of paresis is a sign of damage to the upper motor neurones. These originate in the motor cortex of the brain, pass through an area known as the internal capsule and finally, in the medulla, cross to the opposite side of the body. They then descend down the spinal cord in the pyramidal tracts to reach the anterior horn cells from which the lower motor neurones of the spinal nerves arise.

Damage in the area of the motor cortex by tumour or bleeding may be so limited that the result is a monoparesis, i.e. weakness of a single limb. Damage in the area of the internal capsule in which the fibres are concentrated into only a small area of the brain may lead to a hemiparesis in which the whole of the side of the body opposite to the cerebral lesion is involved. Normally such paresis is often preceded by paralysis, as in a STROKE, but if the causative lesion is a slowly growing tumour paresis may precede true paralysis.

Parkinsonism

The symptoms and signs indicating a derangement of those nerve fibres originating in the brain from the extrapyramidal system.

The chief manifestations of Parkinsonism consist of:

(1) A characteristic TREMOR of the hands which is described as a pill rolling movement.
(2) Rigidity of the muscles which can be demonstrated by attempting to flex the patient's arm. A resistance is encountered which resembles that observed when bending a lead pipe.
(3) Slowness and lack of precision in carrying out movements.

Parkinsonism may be the result of:

(1) Unknown causes. In the majority of sufferers in the United Kingdom there is no known cause although obviously the appropriate nerve pathways are found to have been destroyed.
(2) Viral infection. Between 1916 and 1928 a worldwide epidemic of encephalitis lethargica occurred. Patients who recovered later developed severe Parkinsonism.
(3) Injury. Parkinsonism is common in the punch-drunk boxer who has sustained repeated injury to the

brain leading to tiny HAEMORRHAGES within the brain tissue.

(4) Arterial degeneration. Cerebral atherosclerosis if affecting the blood supply to the extrapyramidal system may lead to this condition.

(5) Chemical agents. The administration of any drug which interferes with the transmission of nerve impulses within the extrapyramidal system may cause Parkinsonism. These include drugs such as methyldopa and the phenothiazines.

Paroxysmal tachycardia

A condition in which intermittent paroxysms of tachycardia occur lasting from a few seconds to a number of hours or even days in which the patient complains of the regular rapid beating of the heart.

The condition may occur in individuals with a completely normal heart in some of whom an attack is precipitated by emotion, exertion, smoking or the excessive consumption of tea or coffee. It may also occur in patients suffering from almost any variety of heart disease.

The precise mechanism is unknown, one explanation is that it is caused by the sudden discharges from an ectopic atrial focus. An attack can often be relieved by pressure on the carotid sinus.

Peau d'orange

This literally means 'orange peel' and is a sign indicating the local obstruction of dermal lymphatics leading to dermal OEDEMA. This sign is usually associated with carcinoma of the breast when infiltration of the local lymphatic channels with malignant disease causes this characteristic appearance of the overlying skin. It may, however, present as a more general appearance, particularly of the lower quadrants of a pendulous breast when the axillary lymphatic nodes have become blocked by metastatic disease.

Peritonitis

Peritonitis or INFLAMMATION of the peritoneum lining the abdominal cavity has many causes. It may be acute or chronic, bacterial or chemical. Acute peritonitis is usually associated with the perforation of one of the hollow abdominal viscera such as the duodenum, gall bladder, appendix or colon.

The main symptom of peritonitis is pain which is severe and constant and it is limited to the area of the abdomen overlying the inflamed parietal peritoneum. The following signs suggest the diagnosis:

(1) A fixed abdomen, showing little if any respiratory movement; the patient may have his legs drawn up to fix the abdominal muscles.
(2) Palpation reveals abdominal tenderness, due to the underlying inflammation, and board-like rigidity, due to spasm of the abdominal muscle.
(3) REBOUND TENDERNESS. When the palpating hand is withdrawn gently from the abdominal wall, the patient experiences a sudden increase in pain.
(4) PARALYTIC ILEUS, seen only after the condition has become established.
(5) FEVER.
(6) Raised pulse rate.
(7) The 'Hippocratic' facies in which the temples are hollow, the eyes sunken and the eyelids slightly parted with the eyes glazed.
(8) In the late stages a combination of hypovolaemic and toxic SHOCK.

The profound systemic effects of peritonitis are due to the rapid absorption of bacterial toxins from the large surface involved. In bacterial peritonitis the organisms most commonly involved are the bacteria of the gastrointestinal tract which include the 'coliforms' together with the anaerobic bacteroides. Less commonly the pneumococci, gonococci or *Mycobacterium tuberculosis* are involved.

Peutz–Jegher's syndrome

A syndrome in which diffuse polyposis of the small intestine occurs in association with facial and buccal pigmentation. This condition is inherited. The polyps do not become malignant and the disorder usually presents with recurrent attacks of abdominal pain due to intermittent intussusception occurring.

Phantom limb

A symptom consisting of a persistent and sometimes disabling pain felt in the non-existent limb following amputation, for which there is no satisfactory physiological explanation. The affected patient is able, very accurately, to localize precisely the area in which the pain is felt. He may remark that it is in the heel or toes. Phantom pain is more common after major than minor amputations.

Phenylketonuria

A sign that an INBORN ERROR OF METABOLISM has occurred associated with a disturbance of the metabolism of the amino acid, phenylalanine. An affected infant may make apparently normal progress or be troubled by persistent VOMITING. Anxiety is aroused by the slow emotional and neurological development when the child reaches approximately 8 to 10 months.

An untreated infant develops into a physically sound but mentally defective adult with minimal signs of neurological abnormality. The diagnosis can be made by various screening tests. Should the test be positive, the immediate treatment should be a phenylalanine-free diet. If this is done at an early stage, brain damage will be avoided.

Photophobia

Intolerance to light. Photophobia may be due to a variety of causes:

(1) Irritative lesions of the eye, including conjunctivitis, corneal injury or INFLAMMATION and iritis.
(2) Excessive exposure of the eyes to ultraviolet rays which is usually caused by failure to protect the eyes with

152

proper filters and may occur in the course of snow skiing, welding with an electric arc or even during sun-bathing. Such photophobia is usually associated with pain in the eyes.

(3) ALBINISM.
(4) HYSTERIA.
(5) Migraine.
(6) Ophthalmic herpes.
(7) Cerebral irritation, e.g. meningitis.

Pickwickian syndrome

A condition characterized by somnolence in an obese patient. The syndrome is named after a Dickensian character described in *The Pickwick Papers*. Such an individual suffers from a chronically raised carbon dioxide level in the blood, mild hypnoxia and polycythaemia. Unlike a normal individual in whom an elevation of the carbon dioxide concentration causes wakefulness, such patients are insensitive to this stimulus and respond only to a further lowering of the oxygen tension in the blood. Characteristically sleep is interrupted by an abrupt waking with snorting respiration. The cause of this peculiar syndrome is usually a disorder of the brain stem, although it is occasionally seen in overweight babies.

Pigmentation, shin see SHIN PIGMENTATION

Pink puffer syndrome

A syndrome observed in the patient suffering from emphysema which is characterized by the permanent over-inflation of the distal air spaces of the lungs occurring in the later stages of the disease. The principal symptom is increasing breathlessness on exertion with increasingly severe attacks of DYSPNOEA should a respiratory tract infection occur.

Inspection reveals a distended, barrel-shaped chest fixed in the inspiration position. Expansion and inspiration can therefore only be achieved with the aid of the accessory muscles. Expiration because of the associated difficulties is unduly prolonged and is often accompanied by pursing of the lips.

If chronic bronchitis has not led to difficulty in the gaseous exchange, the patient remains well oxygenated (therefore of a good colour), although hyperventilating and dyspnoeic, hence the term, pink puffer.

Pneumaturia

A sign of fistula formation between the bladder and a hollow viscus in which air is passed per urethra during micturition.

The common causes include diverticulitis of the pelvic colon when this symptom is usually intermittent, carcinoma of the colon when this symptom becomes progressively worse and rarely, Crohn's disease of either the small or large bowel.

Pneumothorax

The presence of air in the pleural cavity. A pneumothorax may be:

(1) Therapeutic. In the pre-antibiotic era tuberculous infection of the lungs was frequently treated by the induction of an artificial pneumothorax. Air was introduced into the pleural cavity to cause partial collapse of the affected lung. This 'rested' the affected lung, allowing it to heal.

(2) Operative. Any operation which involves opening the pleural cavity is followed by the admission of air and collapse of the lung because its natural elasticity causes it to shrink in the presence of normal atmospheric pressure. Such air is usually removed at the end of the operation by inserting an 'underwater' drain into the chest. This permits air to leave the chest during expiration and prevents its return during inspiration.

(3) Accidental. An injury to the chest which damages the visceral pleura and the underlying lung is liable to be followed by a pneumothorax. Occasionally the opening in the visceral pleura acts as a valve allowing increasing amounts of air to leak into the pleural cavity on inspiration but closing on expiration. Air rapidly accumulates in the affected pleural space, collapse of the lung on the affected side occurs together with displacement of the heart and great vessels to the opposite side of the chest. As first one lung then the other collapses increasing respiratory distress follows. This condition, known

154

as a tension pneumothorax, requires urgent treatment by the immediate introduction of a wide-bore needle into the chest in order to decrease the intrapleural pressure.

(4) Pathological or spontaneous. A spontaneous pneumothorax may be a sign of:

(a) A minor congenital defect in the wall of a subpleural alveolus. If such an alveolus should burst a spontaneous pneumothorax develops usually accompanied by sudden pleuritic pain and DYSPNOEA.

(b) In middle age and after patients suffering from chronic bronchitis and emphysema may rupture an alveolus by coughing.

(c) Any inflammatory conditions such as tuberculosis or staphylococcal pneumonia may occasionally be followed by a spontaneous pneumothorax.

The effect of any type of pneumothorax depends largely on the volume of air and the rapidity with which the air gains access to the pleural cavity. Large volumes cause collapse of the lung on the affected side and movement of the mediastinum towards the unaffected side. This may severely embarrass the action of the heart, particularly in elderly patients who are already suffering from cardiac ischaemia and ANGINA.

Pontine syndrome

A group of clinical syndromes caused by a variety of lesions in the pontine area of the brain such as HAEMORRHAGE or thrombosis of the vascular supply. When the lower pons is involved the origin of the sixth cranial nerve which innervates the external rectus muscle of the eye is destroyed so that lateral rotation of the eye on the affected side, together with a hemiplegia on the opposite side of the body occurs. Since the seventh nerve nucleus is very close to this area, it too may be involved leading to a facial palsy on the side of the lesion.

Disease in other areas of the pons causes a wide variety of different syndromes because of the large number of separate nerve centres in this part of the brain.

Porphyria

An uncommon inherited group of diseases in which the metabolism of pigments known as the porphyrins is abnormal. These chemical compounds are manufactured during the formation of the haem pigment of haemoglobin.

Many varieties of porphyria exist with somewhat different characteristics. In one group a chronic eczema of the skin occurs when it is exposed to light, whereas in another variety intermittent acute ABDOMINAL PAIN, neuritis and DELIRIUM occur. The reasons for these various manifestations are quite unknown.

Portal hypertension

A sign of increased pressure within the portal system of veins which drain the gastrointestinal tract.

The increase in pressure may be caused by:

(1) Thrombosis of the portal vein.
(2) Diseases of the liver such as cirrhosis.
(3) Obstruction of the hepatic veins draining liver blood into the inferior vena cava.
(4) Right-sided heart failure when back pressure on the portal system occurs.

The various clinical signs of portal hypertension include:

(1) The development of extensive collaterals in areas in which the systemic and portal systems communicate. This causes oesophageal varices, haemorrhoids and the CAPUT MEDUSAE. By developing collaterals the blood of the splanchnic area can be returned to the heart without passing through the liver.
(2) Splenic enlargement due in part to venous congestion but also to hyperplasia. The latter may lead to the condition of hypersplenism and ANAEMIA.
(3) ASCITES which is due to a combination of factors including:
   (a) Impairment of protein production in severe liver disease.
   (b) Excessive circulation of the hormone aldosterone,

which retains sodium and, therefore, water in the circulation.

(4) HEPATIC ENCEPHALOPATHY.

Post-concussional syndrome

A group of symptoms which may follow a relatively trivial head injury. The symptoms include HEADACHE, dizziness, ANXIETY, various fears, lassitude and irritability. The cause is really unknown although it can nearly always be assumed that minor degrees of brain damage have preceded the onset of the syndrome.

Projectile vomiting

A symptom of effortless VOMITING, the vomitus being ejected over a considerable distance.

It is commonly seen in babies suffering from congenital hypertrophic pyloric stenosis and less commonly in adults suffering from duodenal ulceration associated with severe scarring or cancer of the pyloric antrum leading to stenosis. Less often projectile vomiting may be seen in certain cerebral conditions such as meningitis.

Proteinuria

The presence of excessive quantities of protein in the urine. Protein can be detected in the urine by the use of an Albustix (Ames Co.) which is roughly quantitative, giving an indication of the amount of protein present. A second test is to boil the urine after acidifying it with acetic acid which prevents the precipitation of phosphate. The development of a white cloud in the urine denotes the presence of protein which has been coagulated by the heat.

Normally the quantity of protein which escapes from the kidney is too small to be detected by either of these methods but should the glomeruli be damaged as in glomerulo-nephritis, protein leaks from the renal capillaries into the tubules and appears in the urine. This loss of protein, especially albumin, may reach as much as 20 to 30 g a day. Losses of 10 g a day or more lead to such a fall in the albumin concentration in the plasma that the osmotic pressure of the plasma decreases. The result is that fluid forced out from the arterial side of a capillary by hydrostatic pressure cannot be drawn back into the circulation on the venous side. This fluid remains in the tissues, causing OEDEMA and it is the principal reason why patients suffering from sub-acute nephritis become oedematous.

Pruritis

An intense itching, causing a desire to scratch or rub the skin. Pruritis may be mild and intermittent, related to changes in body temperature, local or general, and occasionally so intense as to make the patient suicidal.

The sensation of itching probably travels from the skin to the spinal cord and onwards to the brain in the same nerve fibres that carry pain sensation. In the skin itself it is possible that the nerve endings are stimulated by a variety of chemical substances. These include histamine, bile salts and enzymes responsible for breaking down protein.

Pruritis may be a symptom of many conditions including:

(1) Psychological disturbance, especially in the neurotic or depressed patient, is commonly associated with pruritis ani or vulvi.

(2) Local diseases of the skin including:

   (a) Infestations with parasites such as scabies, pediculus or fleas.

   (b) URTICARIA, psoriasis, eczema, seborrhoeic dermatitis and lichen planus.

   (c) If areas of the skin which are normally dry become bathed in abnormal secretions, pruritis often follows. Thus pruritis may be the presenting symptom of haemorrhoids or a vaginal discharge.

(3) General diseases:

   (a) Obstructive jaundice is often associated with generalized itching which is caused by the accumulation of bile salts in the blood. Removal of the obstruction is normally followed by immediate relief.

(b) Hodgkin's and associated diseases of the reticulo-endothelial system.

(c) Diabetes mellitus.

(d) Senility.

Ptosis

A drooping of the upper eyelids. The causes may be congenital, due to maldevelopment of the muscles of the upper eyelid when it is often associated with a squint, or acquired.

Acquired ptosis may be a sign of:

(1) PARALYSIS of the third cranial oculomotor nerve. Unilateral paralysis is rare but occurs in diseases affecting the cavernous sinus, such as cavernous sinus thrombosis. Bilateral third nerve palsy follows lesions involving the mid-brain such as haemorrhage or tumours.

　　If the third nerve is the only one affected, which is rare, ptosis, together with external rotation of the eye due to the unopposed action of the sixth cranial nerve, results and the pupil also dilates due to the unopposed action of the sympathetic fibres.

(2) Destruction of the cervical sympathetic nervous system due to direct involvement by tumours of the neck or injuries which involve the brachial plexus. Such lesions are associated with ptosis, slight retraction of the eyeball (meiosis) and constriction of the pupil due to the unopposed action of the parasympathetic nervous system. This is HORNER'S SYNDROME.

(3) The levator muscle of the eyelid is commonly affected in myasthenia gravis, a condition in which the function of the neuromuscular junction is disorganized even though it remains normal in appearance. The disease, affecting women more commonly than men, frequently presents with ptosis and DIPLOPIA due to the involvement of the extra-ocular muscles.

Pulsus alternans

A sign of severe left ventricular failure in which the pulse beats are evenly spaced in time but are alternatively large and small in volume. This type of pulse may be detected by palpating the radial pulse or observing changes in the peripheral blood pressure. The mechanism whereby this type of pulse is caused is unknown.

Pulsus paradoxus

The marked diminution of the radial pulse during inspiration; a sign of cardiac compression caused either by a pericardial effusion or constrictive pericarditis both of which interfere with myocardial function by reducing the input of blood and therefore the output of the heart.

In a normal individual slight alterations in the volume of the pulse occur during the inspiratory phase because of the increasingly negative intrathoracic pressure which develops. This leads to a temporary increase in the volume of blood within the pulmonary vessels which are dilated during this phase of respiration. Temporarily, therefore, the amount of blood available to the left side of the heart is diminished with a result that the cardiac output decreases and so the peripheral pulse volume declines.

In the presence of a pericardial effusion these natural physiological responses are exaggerated because cardiac function is already disturbed.

Purpura

A haemorrhagic rash which may involve the skin or mucous membranes caused by the extravasation of blood from the capillaries into the surrounding tissues.

These extravasations may vary in size from a pinhead to a large bruise. Purpuric spots which involve the mucous membrane, may take the form of 'blood blisters' or lead to obvious bleeding, e.g. EPISTAXIS, MELAENA, HAEMATURIA or MANORRHAGIA.

Purpura is a sign of:

(1) Deficiency in the number or function of the platelets—THROMBOCYTOPENIA or thrombasthenia. The cause of a thrombocytopenic purpura may be unknown (the condition of idiopathic thrombocytopenic purpura); or it may be due to the development of antibodies which destroy the existing platelets; or lastly it may be secondary to

some other condition suppressing the bone marrow and preventing the production of platelets. Secondary thrombocytopenic purpura occurs in:

(a) Hypoplastic or aplastic ANAEMIA.
(b) Pernicious anaemia.
(c) Leukaemia.
(d) Invasion of the bone marrow by metastases.
(e) Some forms of drug therapy.

(2) Damage to the walls of the capillaries, the result of:

(a) Antibodies—leading to allergic purpura which is often accompanied by URTICARIA, as in the HENOCH–SCHOENLEIN SYNDROME.
(b) Deficiency of vitamin C—SCURVY.
(c) Bacterial toxins.
(d) Metabolic toxins e.g. terminal renal failure, producing URAEMIA is commonly associated with purpura.

(3) Increased mobility of an inelastic skin leading to rupture of small blood vessels. This is seen in the elderly and is known as senile purpura.

The tendency to purpura can sometimes be demonstrated by Hess's test. A sphygmomanometer cuff is inflated to 80 mm Hg and left for approximately 5 minutes. A crop of purpuric spots below the cuff is a positive sign. All forms of purpura are associated with a prolonged BLEEDING TIME.

Pyaemia

Pyaemia denotes the presence in the circulation of infected thrombus. The disintegrating thrombus is carried to various organs where it produces metastatic ABSCESSES or septic infarcts. The common causative lesions of a pyaemia are carbuncle, osteomyelitis and puerperal sepsis; these cause the development of pyaemic lung abscesses. Uncontrolled infection in the gastrointestinal tract such as acute appendicitis leads to a portal pyaemia and multiple abscesses in the liver.

The symptoms associated with a pyaemia are principally due to the original infection and the site of the subsequent metastatic abscesses. However, in the majority of cases irregular RIGORS occur.

Pyuria

The presence of pus cells in the urine. Pus cells usually indicate the presence of renal, vesical, prostatic or urethral infection.

In the majority of patients the chief symptom associated with pyuria is DYSURIA and culture of the urine will yield a significant growth of organisms. If the culture is sterile despite the presence of many pus cells a search must be made for the *Mycobacterium tuberculosis* which can only be grown on special media.

Raynaud's phenomenon

A condition in which the digital arteries supplying the fingers with blood are abnormally sensitive to cold.

Exposed to cold the fingers undergo a series of colour changes, first white, then slowly becoming blue and, as attack terminates, red, hot and painful. These various changes are caused by contraction of the digital arteries, stagnation of blood in the dilated capillaries and finally a relaxation of the constricted arteries and arterioles which leads to an increased blood flow through the tissues.

Raynaud's phenomenon is most commonly a sign of:

(1) Atherosclerosis.
(2) Collagen diseases.
(3) Cervical rib.
(4) Prolonged exposure of the hands to excessive vibration.

When the same vascular phenomena occur without apparent cause the condition is termed Raynaud's disease. When the condition is severe, GANGRENE of the terminal digits may follow an attack.

Rebound tenderness

A sign of irritation, most commonly the result of INFLAMMATION, of the parietal peritoneum.

Rebound tenderness is, therefore, found in association with general PERITONITIS from whatever cause, over an inflamed viscus such as an acutely inflamed appendix or over a strangulated length of bowel.

It occurs due to reflex spasm of the abdominal muscles which

162

contract in response to the intense PAIN caused by the sudden movement of the sensitive parietal peritoneum as the palpating fingers are removed from the abdominal wall.

Referred pain

Pain caused by pathological changes in an organ which is interpreted by the sufferer as cutaneous in origin. Examples of referred pain include the pain of cardiac ischaemia which is often felt in the arms, and pain which is felt in the neck and shoulder which arises from disease of the diaphragmatic pleura.

The various explanations which have been advanced for the mechanism by which visceral pain is referred to different parts of the body have altered with our increasing knowledge of neurophysiology. At present the accepted explanation is as follows.

Impulses from a diseased viscus such as the heart travel via the fibres of the sympathetic nervous system through the appropriate dorsal (posterior) nerve root and into the spinal cord. In the dorsal horn these fibres become the near neighbours of pain fibres subserving sensation from a particular part of the skin and subcutaneous tissues. Normally at this point a synapse occurs with the second order neurone which crosses the cord and passes upwards in the spinothalamic tracts to the brain. Because, however, there are more incoming fibres in the dorsal root than there are nerve fibres in the ascending tracts of the spinal cord it is obvious that some congestion must occur and that some fibres from the heart and from the superficial tissues must synapse with the same ascending fibres. As a result a visceral impulse reaching the brain may be incorrectly interpreted as an impulse from the skin, so causing the individual to complain of pain of cutaneous distribution.

Reflex

Examination of the various reflexes of the body is extremely helpful in the diagnosis of neurological disease. Those commonly examined include:

(1) The deep or tendon reflexes; examples of which include the biceps, triceps and supinator jerks of the upper limb and the knee and ankle jerks of the lower limbs.

(2) The superficial or cutaneous reflexes, examples of which include the plantar reflex of the foot (BABINSKI'S SIGN), the epigastric reflexes of the abdomen and the cremaster reflex of the thigh.

(3) Cilio-spinal reflex, involving the pupillary reaction to light.

In addition other reflexes are important to the body's proper function including the micturition and defaecation reflexes, each concerned with the act described but capable of modification by the higher centres of the brain.

For a reflex to be present it is necessary for a stimulus to be carried in the appropriate sensory nerve, reach the spinal cord and then be immediately relayed to the appropriate motor neurones. In the case of the deep tendon reflexes the sensory stimulus consists of a brief stretching of the appropriate muscle, e.g. to elicit the knee jerk the patellar tendon is tapped with a hammer which results in an involuntary stretching of the quadriceps muscle, a sensory impulse then travels via the fourth lumbar nerve to the spinal cord and immediately stimulates the motor nerve supplying the quadriceps muscle. The result is a short but rapid contraction.

The presence of a normal reflex indicates that the particular part of the spinal cord concerned with the reflex is functioning in a proper manner. However, each reflex can be modified by impulses carried down the spinal cord by descending nerve tracts arising in the brain and brain stem. Thus when the descending tracts are damaged by disease or injury an exaggerated hyperactive type of reflex occurs. Thus in a patient suffering from a STROKE accompanied by PARESIS exaggerated tendon reflexes will be found on the affected side. Although the tendon reflexes are exaggerated the superficial or cutaneous reflexes are in fact abolished in similar circumstances.

A reflex is, of course, lost altogether when either the afferent (sensory) nerve, the spinal centre in which the sensory and motor nerves meet or the motor nerves themselves are damaged or destroyed by injury or disease.

Reiter's syndrome

A combination of urethritis, arthritis, conjunctivitis and dysentery.

The arthritis is often the dominant feature. It is non-suppurative and tends to involve the peripheral joints of the lower limbs, together with the sacroiliac joints. Although believed to be of infectious origin, no infective agent has yet been isolated.

Retention of urine

An inability to empty the bladder. Retention may be acute or chronic. In acute retention the distension of the bladder occurs so rapidly that it causes considerable discomfort or even pain in the lower abdomen. In chronic retention the bladder distends over a much longer period and the vesical muscle atrophies and is unable to contract. Chronic retention is, therefore, painless and is nearly always associated with incontinence as the urine dribbles through the overstretched internal urethral sphincter.

Retention is a symptom of many different conditions and these may be classified as follows:

(1) Mechanical obstruction to the outflow of urine:
  (a) In males:
    (i) Enlargement of prostate, benign or malignant.
    (ii) Traumatic or inflammatory strictures of the urethra.
    (iii) Stenosis of the urethral meatus or prepuce.
    (iv) Carcinoma involving the bladder outlet.
    (v) Stone in the bladder.
  (b) In females:
    (i) Bladder outlet obstruction caused by the enlarging uterus of pregnancy or uterine fibroids.
    (ii) Carcinoma of bladder.
(2) Neurogenic conditions:
  (a) Spinal shock. An injury to the vertebral column causing acute spinal cord damage in either sex is ini-

tially associated with retention of urine, due to the immediate separation of the bladder from the higher centres of the brain. Since this separation includes severance of the sensory pathways to the brain the retention is painless, even though it is acute.

(b) Injury to the autonomic ganglia in the pelvis which supply the motor nerves of the bladder muscle. Injuries of this type are nearly always caused by pelvic surgery such as abdomino-perineal resection of rectum or radical hysterectomy.

(c) Occurring as a complication of diseases which affect the spinal cord such as multiple sclerosis, poliomyelitis or tabes dorsalis.

(3) Reflex. Retention of urine commonly occurs in individuals subjected to painful conditions or operations in the immediate vicinity of the urethra, thus acute retention may occur following haemorrhoidectomy or childbirth. Retention of this type is particularly prone to occur in males suffering some degree of prostatic enlargement.

(4) FUNCTIONAL conditions. HYSTERIA may be associated with retention.

Retrosternal pain

A common symptom of oesophageal disease caused by a combination of muscular spasm and superficial ulceration of the lining mucous membrane. Both most frequently occur in the presence of a hiatus hernia in which condition the gastric juice is able to reflux into the lower oesophagus causing mucosal INFLAMMATION. This type of retrosternal pain, known as HEARTBURN, is provoked by stooping or by lying in the horizontal position.

Retrosternal pain may also be caused by cardiac ischaemia or a myocardial infarct. In either case the pain is described as griping or choking in character and frequently radiates into the neck and down the arm.

Rhinorrhoea, cerebrospinal see CEREBROSPINAL RHINORRHOEA

Rice-water stools

The characteristic stool passed by the cholera victim after an incubation period of 2 to 4 days. The stool is a thin fluid, greyish-white in colour, containing flecks of mucus, the latter giving rise to the classic descriptive phrase. In severe cholera the volume of the stools may reach 17 litres/24 hours, so that large quantities of sodium, potassium and water are lost with the result that hypokalaemia and DEHYDRATION develop with great rapidity.

Rice-water stools are also seen in patients suffering from pseudomembranous enterocolitis, a condition which may occasionally occur following the administration of antibiotics which alter the bacterial flora of the gut. In the commonest variety the gut becomes infected with an antibiotic-resistant *Staphylococcus*. This condition has become rarer as the so-called prophylactic use of antibiotics to prevent post-operative wound sepsis has fallen into disfavour.

Rigor

A rigor is a severe uncontrollable shivering attack attended by a sudden elevation of the temperature and marked rise in pulse rate.

A rigor may be caused by:
(1) Specific infections:
    (a) Bacterial, e.g. catheter fever, acute cholecystitis, cholangitis or acute pyelonephritis.
    (b) Viral. e.g. virus pneumonia.
    (c) Plasmodial, e.g. malaria.
(2) The administration of therapeutic sera such as anti-tetanus toxoid which is derived from horse serum containing toxin treated with formaldehyde.
(3) A mis-matched blood transfusion in which rapid destruction of the donor cells occurs.

A rigor is the first part of a 3-stage reaction by the body to these various causes. In the first stage known as the cold stage the patient feels intensely cold and begins to shiver. The internal temperature of the body rises but the skin temperature remains inappropriately low due to vasoconstriction of the blood vessels of the skin, with the result that the heat formed in the body cannot be lost by the evaporation of sweat or by convection but only by conduction. This mechanism is insufficient to prevent the temperature from rising abruptly so that the patient enters a second stage known as the hot stage. In this the patient ceases to shiver and begins to feel distressingly hot. The skin becomes flushed, dry and warm and the patient becomes restless or even delirious. During this stage the temperature may reach 40°C. In the third and last stage profuse sweating occurs followed by a dramatic fall in the body temperature.

Risus sardonicus

The mocking or sneering facial expression of a patient suffering from tetanus which is caused by spasm of the facial muscles. This causes the central portion of the mouth to be pulled upwards and the corners downwards and outwards. Risus sardonicus is nearly always associated with TRISMUS.

Rombergism

A sign of central nervous system disease affecting those nerve fibres in the spinal cord which carry the sensations concerned with position of the joints and the tone of the controlling muscles. This is collectively known as proprioceptive sensation. These nerve fibres after reaching the spinal cord via the peripheral nerves, enter the dorsal column.

Abolition of proprioceptive sensation causes ATAXIA which is usually worse in the dark because, when such an individual is unable to see, he cannot relate his limbs to his surroundings by the normal visual aids.

To test for Rombergism the patient is requested to stand erect with his eyes closed. In the presence of disease affecting the dorsal column, the patient gradually begins to sway and may eventually fall forwards. This is known as a positive Romberg sign.

Diseases which affect the dorsal column of the spinal cord and thus lead to Rombergism and ataxia include syphilis of the central nervous system and vitamin B_{12} deficiency.

Sabre tibiae

A sign rarely seen at the present day in which the anterior borders of the tibiae become prominent due to an INFLAMMA-TION of the periosteum by the causative organism of syphilis, the *Treponema pallidum*.

Sciatica

A symptom complex rather than a disease which is due to irritation of the roots of the sciatic nerve or the nerve itself.

Although commonly caused by pressure from a lumbar disc on a nerve root it may also be the result of other conditions such as spinal tumours, pelvic tumours or spondylolisthesis if the appropriate nerves are irritated or invaded.

Sciatic pain due to disc pressure on the fifth lumbar nerve usually causes low back pain and pain in the buttock which then passes down the thigh to the calf or heel. Numbness or PARESTHESIAE may occur together with muscle weakness and loss of tendon jerks.

In an acute attack the patient is commonly unable to flex the spine and a lumbar SCOLIOSIS may be present in which the curvature of the spine is either towards or away from the protruding disc depending upon the exact point at which it irritates the nerve root.

Scoliosis

When viewed from the back any deviation from the normally straight spine to one side or the other, that is a lateral deviation, constitutes scoliosis.

The presence of scoliosis is evidence of a variety of pathological conditions. In young girls it may merely be evidence of bad posture when the curve is usually slight, single and frequently with its concavity to the right. Such a curve disappears in recumbency or when the child hangs from a bar. In this type there is no structural abnormality of the spine. Structural scoliosis may be idiopathic, that is of unknown origin, or due to congenital or acquired disease of the vertebral column or to disease of the muscles which support the spine.

A common cause of structural scoliosis in the past, was poliomyelitis in which PARALYSIS of the muscles supporting the spine frequently occurred. A less common cause was an actual anomaly of the vertebral column itself.

Scurvy

A sign of a deficiency of vitamin C (ascorbic acid). The main function of this vitamin is to maintain collagen formation in the connective tissues. If this is not properly formed, the endothelium of the capillaries and smaller blood vessels tends to disintegrate and bleeding occurs. In the presence of a deficiency of vitamin C changes in the bones also occur, the conversion of calcified cartilage to bone being delayed and because calcified cartilage is more brittle fractures are common.

Vitamin C deficiency in a child causes irritability, ANAEMIA, subperiosteal HAEMATOMAS and enlargement of the costochondral junctions, the 'rickety rosary'.

In an adult there may be few symptoms in the early stages, but as the deficiency becomes worse, if the patient still possesses his own teeth, the gums become swollen, bluish in colour and bleed. In both adults and infants spontaneous internal bleeding may occur.

Septicaemia

A sign that large numbers of pathogenic bacteria are present and multiplying in the blood stream of an individual whose defence mechanisms against bacterial invasion have been overwhelmed.

The symptoms and signs of septicaemia include FEVER, RIGORS, TACHYCARDIA and increased respiratory rate. The patient may VOMIT, suffer DIARRHOEA and because of the tremendous loss of fluid, rapidly become DEHYDRATED. When bacterial invasion of the liver occurs, the patient becomes CACHECTIC and JAUNDICED.

Sheehan's syndrome

A syndrome consisting of myxoedema, AMENORRHOEA, loss of libido, depression and apathy resulting from a deficiency of the pituitary hormones. This is usually caused by thrombosis of the arterial supply of the gland following a post-partum haemorrhage.

170

Shin pigmentation

One of the commoner causes of shin pigmentation is the deposition of haemosiderin in the subcutaneous tissues. This pigment is derived from haemoglobin liberated from erythrocytes which have escaped into the tissues from the capillaries. Such pigmentation is usually accompanied by thickening of the underlying subcutaneous tissues and in some patients active ULCERATION of the skin.

The underlying pathology is a damaged deep venous system in the leg of such severity that it has led to destruction of the valves in this system. In the presence of an incompetent valvular mechanism the venous pressure in the calf is equal to the vertical height between the leg and the right atrium and this instead of falling, as it does in a normal leg on exercise, actually rises because the so-called 'leg muscle pump' becomes inefficient.

As a result the pressure rises in those capillaries connected to the perforating veins and so erythrocytes escape into the tissues. The eventual thickening of the subcutaneous tissues is due to their reaction to the haemosiderin and the ulceration to increasing local ANOXIA.

Pigmentation of this type should be distinguished from that caused by the chronic applications of heat, a condition not uncommon in the aged who may sit for long periods in front of a fire.

Shock

A term used to describe a clinical syndrome in which one of the most important features is a fall in BLOOD PRESSURE.

The causes of shock include:

(1) A sudden reduction in the volume of fluid in the circulation—hypovolaemic shock which may be caused by:

    (a) The loss of whole blood, as in haemorrhage from a wound or a bleeding duodenal ulcer.

    (b) A loss of plasma, as in severe burns or acute pancreatitis.

    (c) A loss of water and salt from the body due to severe VOMITING or DIARRHOEA.

171

A sudden reduction in the volume of fluid in the circulation causes a diminishing volume of blood to return to the right side of the heart and hence a diminished cardiac output from the left side. This results in a fall in the systemic blood pressure. The pressure sensors in the great vessels known as the baroreceptors monitor this fall and as a result of reflex action via the autonomic nervous system and the vasomotor centre in the brain stem the following compensatory changes take place in order to diminish the harmful effects which may particularly damage the brain and kidneys:

(a) The venous side of the circulation, which normally holds about three-quarters of the total blood volume, contracts. This action can temporarily restore the effective blood volume and so increase the volume of blood returning to the heart.

(b) The peripheral arterioles contract and by increasing the peripheral resistance raise the blood pressure to more normal levels.

These compensatory mechanisms may be highly effective. A healthy adult male suffers a fall in blood pressure for only about 2 hours after losing one litre of blood. Losses larger than this, however, are greater than the compensatory mechanisms can cope with. A loss of 2 litres of blood leads to a fall in the systolic blood pressure to 65 mmHg or less. Persistence of such a low pressure will eventually lead to renal damage.

(2) The heart ceases to act as an efficient pump—cardiogenic shock. In consequence the output of blood from the heart falls accompanied by a declining blood pressure. The commonest cause of cardiogenic shock is severe myocardial infarction.

The action of the heart may also be grossly disturbed if the venous return is suddenly reduced. This is occasionally caused by a massive pulmonary embolus which is so large that the pulmonary arteries are completely obstructed.

(3) The peripheral circulation is disrupted. Dilatation,

paralysis or destruction of the arterioles and capillaries effectively reduces the circulating blood volume because blood is retained within them and in addition fluid leaks from the circulation into the surrounding tissues. This state may be caused by a variety of factors including:

(a) Bacterial endotoxins causing endotoxic or bacteraemic shock. These toxins destroy the smaller blood vessels.

(b) ANAPHYLAXIS, causing anaphylactic shock. The antigen–antibody reaction associated with anaphylaxis causes the release of a number of chemical substances one of which is known as histamine. This not only paralyses the peripheral circulation but also increases its permeability and so allows protein and fluid to escape from the circulation.

(c) Nervous influences causing neurogenic shock. Any noxious nervous influence such as emotion, spinal cord injury or spinal anaesthesia, may be followed by such a loss of sympathetic vasomotor tone that the arterioles dilate and the peripheral resistance falls.

Apart from the fall in blood pressure the signs and symptoms of shock vary somewhat with the cause but usually include:

(1) An increase in heart rate due to the action of nervous impulses arising from the pressure sensors, known as baroreceptors in the great vessels.

(2) Thready pulse; due to the reduced cardiac output causing a reduced pulse pressure.

(3) Cold extremities due to the peripheral constriction or diminished blood flow through the peripheral circulation.

Shoulder-tip pain

Excluding local conditions of the shoulder itself, shoulder-tip pain is more frequently a REFERRED PAIN indicating disease of the diaphragmatic pleura, or alternatively of the parietal peritoneum below the diaphragm. Disease in these areas causes pain in the shoulders because the diaphragm receives both its sensory and motor supply from the third, fouth and fifth cervical segments, segments which also supply the sensory cutaneous nerves to the tip of the shoulder.

The physician will hear of the complaint of shoulder-tip pain in patients suffering from diaphragmatic pleurisy, and the surgeon, from patients suffering from perforated duodenal ULCERATION when the acid gastric contents irritate.

Sinus

A tract leading from an ABSCESS deep in the tissues to the surface. If a sinus is persistent there must be an underlying cause. For example, a pilonidal sinus occurring between the buttocks usually contains a collection of hairs. These have been driven or sucked through the skin and, lying in the subcutaneous tissues, provoke a continuing inflammatory response. Another example of an intractable sinus is that which follows infection of a surgical wound when non-absorbable suture material has been buried within it. A sinus must be distinguished from a FISTULA which is a tract connecting two hollow viscera or a hollow viscus and the surface.

The term sinus is also used to describe:

(1) The cavities in the facial bones which are filled with air.
(2) Various blood vessels such as the coronary sinus in which blood is returned from the cardiac muscle to the right atrium, and the venous sinuses lying within the cranium.
(3) Sinus rhythm, the normal rhythm of the heart beat.

Sjögren's syndrome

A condition in which gradual dryness of the eyes and/or mouth occurs in association with rheumatoid ARTHRITIS. Lack of tears causes a burning sensation in the eyes and the patient is unable to protect them from dust, so that corneal ULCERATION may occur. Dryness of the mouth causes difficulty in swallowing and is usually followed by INFLAMMATION and dental caries. The underlying pathology is a chronic inflammation of the lacrimal and salivary glands. A number of antibodies have been found in the blood which react, in particular with salivary duct epithelium, but their precise importance is uncertain

174

because similar antibodies can also be found in many patients suffering from uncomplicated rheumatoid arthritis.

Slough

A sign of underlying ULCERATION, a slough consists of a layer of exudate and dead tissue which lies on the surface of the ulcer. At first the slough is adherent to the underlying granulation tissue but it slowly separates as the undersurface is digested by enzymes. The character of the slough may give a clue to the underlying cause of the ulceration; classically, for example, the slough of a tertiary syphilitic ulcer is likened to a piece of washleather.

Smoky urine

A sign of HAEMATURIA. Uniform discoloration of the urine must be distinguished from other causes, including the ingestion of beetroot or drugs such as phenolphthalein.

Splenomegaly

Splenomegaly or enlargement of the spleen seldom causes symptoms and its presence is usually discovered during the course of an abdominal examination. It may occur alone or in combination with enlargement of the liver.

The following are the commoner causes of moderate splenic enlargement:

(1) Disease of the haemopoietic system such as chronic lymphatic leukaemia, thalassaemia and congenital spherocytosis.
(2) The reticuloses, including the various types of lymphoma and Hodgkin's disease.
(3) Vascular conditions including splenic infarction, splenic vein thrombosis or obstruction.
(4) Cysts of the spleen, the commonest cause of which is an infection by the parasite causing hydatid disease.

Giant enlargement in which the spleen extends beyond the umbilicus occurs in the following conditions:

(1) Diseases of the haemopoietic system such as chronic myeloid leukaemia and polycythaemia.

(2) Infective conditions including chronic malaria, kala azar and tuberculosis.

(3) Congestion of the spleen due to portal vein obstruction.

(4) Massive solitary cysts.

Apart from the presence of a dull ache in the left upper abdomen the symptoms associated with splenomegaly are always those of the causative disease. Thus portal vein obstruction leading to splenomegaly is usually the result of cirrhosis and may, therefore, be associated with the symptoms and signs of chronic liver failure.

Steatorrhoea

An excess of fat in the stools. A patient suffering from steatorrhoea usually complains of the passage of an excessive number of bulky, pale, offensive, unformed stools which tend to float in the lavatory pan. Steatorrhoea is, therefore, a specific form of DIARRHOEA.

The diagnosis may be obvious from an examination of the stools which may be pale and greasy; examined under a microscope, after suitable staining for fat, the globules may be apparent. Absolute measurement of fat absorption can be carried out in a number of different ways. Normally approximately 96 per cent of the fat intake is absorbed so that the intestinal loss is no more than 4 per cent. A loss greater than 7 per cent is regarded as abnormal.

Such excessive fat loss may follow a large variety of conditions.

(1) The absorption of fat depends first on the proper breakdown of the fat in the diet. This is achieved by the action of pancreatic lipase and if this is absent the breakdown of fat cannot occur. Diseases leading to absence of pancreatic lipase include diseases affecting the pancreas as a whole, such as chronic pancreatitis and mucoviscidosis. More commonly, however, lipase is absent because it cannot gain entrance into the duodenum due to obstruction of the pancreatic duct caused by malignant disease in the head of the gland.

(2) The digested fat must then be absorbed and this depends

upon the formation of combinations of bile salts with the products of digestion to produce chemical structures known as micelles. If bile salts are absent these cannot be formed and fat absorption suffers. Steatorrhoea therefore occurs in obstructive jaundice in which condition the bile salts do not gain entrance to the small intestine. Even when bile salts gain entrance to the bowel they may be destroyed by the action of bacteria. This is believed to be the cause of steatorrhoea in conditions such as the 'blind loop syndrome', multiple jejunal diverticuli and partial intestinal obstruction.

(3) Absorption also depends upon a normal length of small bowel from which absorption can occur, a normal intestinal mucosa and a normal rate of transit of the small bowel contents through the gut. The first factor is disturbed if extensive bowel resections have been performed, for example, because of intestinal strangulation. The second factor is disturbed by mucosal diseases which include Crohn's disease, gluten sensitive enteropathy, tropical sprue or tuberculous infection. The third factor is altered by bowel resection or by general diseases such as thyrotoxicosis.

Stokes–Adams attack

A sign of cardiac disease. The patient suddenly becomes pale, pulseless and unconscious due to cerebral ANOXIA which is the result of a sudden diminution in the cardiac output. This may be caused by a sudden change from incomplete to complete HEART BLOCK or by CARDIAC ARREST.

During this type of attack twitching or convulsions may occur and the pupils dilate. The attacks, if short-lived, are followed by a return of consciousness accompanied by flushing as the blood flows through vessels dilated by the hypoxic stage. An attack lasting more than 3 to 4 minutes is inevitably followed by death due to irreversible cerebral damage.

Strangury

A symptom characterized by a frequent, painful and repetitive desire to pass water. Response to this stimulus usually results in the passage of only a few drops of urine.

Strangury occurs in any condition in which the bladder becomes over-sensitive to distension. The common causes include cystitis from any cause and stone in the bladder.

Striae

Lines or streaks found on the skin after it has been temporarily stretched and the underlying elastic tissue has failed to take up the slack, as for example the striae gravidarum; the stretch marks commonly seen on the abdomen of the post-partum woman. Similar markings may also occur in both men and women who have become excessively OBESE and then reduced weight by intensive dieting.

Striae are also a sign of CUSHING'S SYNDROME in which the circulation of excessive amounts of adrenal hormones causes a rapid accumulation of fat in the face, neck and trunk, although the limbs may remain thin. Associated with this increasing adiposity is a breakdown of protein which not only affects the muscles, but also the connective tissues of the skin causing it to become atrophic. This causes the development of broad, depressed striae, usually red or purple in colour, occurring most commonly on the abdomen, buttocks, thighs and mammary regions.

Stridor

A symptom of obstruction to the free passage of air in the larynx or trachea causing a high-pitched wheeze which is usually loudest during inspiration because the flow of air is fastest during this phase of respiration.

Stridor can occur in both childhood and in the adult. In childhood the commonest cause is an acute INFLAMMATION of the larynx and lay individuals often refer to this as 'croup'. A less common cause in this age group is obstruction of the respiratory passages by an inhaled foreign body such as a pea or bead.

In an adult the common causes of stridor are cancer of the larynx, oedema of the larynx from any cause and external pressure upon the trachea by a goitre.

Stroke

A term which is most frequently used to describe the aftermath of acute brain damage brought about by natural disease.

This includes a variety of conditions:

(1) Sudden bleeding into the brain tissue. This may occur when the blood pressure is raised (HYPERTENSION); when the blood vessels of the brain are weakened by diseases such as atherosclerosis or aneurysm, or when abnormal blood vessels are present in the brain as in brain tumours.

(2) Sudden cessation of the blood flowing to the brain either by thrombosis in an atherosclerotic cerebral artery or by an embolus derived elsewhere in the circulation.

Whereas bleeding may progress, leading to increasing signs of brain damage and finally death, the effects of thrombosis or embolus are at their worst immediately after the incident.

The 'stroke' which follows any of these various causes produces PARALYSIS or PARESIS of the muscles on the side of the body opposite to the involved brain tissue. This is because the motor nerves which descend from the cerebral cortex in the pyramidal tracts cross from one side of the brain stem to the other before passing down the spinal cord to meet the spinal motor nerves.

If recovery occurs the patient is left with exaggerated reflexes on the affected side and when the dominant brain hemisphere, which is usually on the left side, has been involved, one of the most troublesome end results may be APHASIA.

Stupor

A condition of partial insensibility, sometimes accompanied by restlessness of the body and mind, when it is known as DELIRIUM.

Stupor may be a sign of psychological disorder or the result of organic conditions such as severe ANAEMIA, incipient diabetic COMA or intoxication with alcohol.

Delirium is usually associated with fever, toxaemia, injury or some forms of psychological disorder. Delirium tremens, for example, is a form of acute delirium seen in chronic alcoholism in which the affected individual become severely disorientated and suffers from HALLUCINATIONS.

Succussion splash

A sign associated with the retention of excessive quantities of fluid and food debris in the stomach. The splash is elicited by either tapping the epigastrium or shaking the patient from side to side.

Such a splash may be present in a perfectly normal individual following the consumption of large quantities of fluid shortly before examination. If, however, it is some time since the consumption of food and drink the demonstration of a splash indicates that the exit from the stomach has been obstructed and that pyloric stenosis is present.

In an adult the common causes of such stenosis include chronic duodenal ulceration or cancer of the pyloric end of the stomach. If either condition remains unrelieved ALKALOSIS and CACHEXIA soon follow. In an infant pyloric stenosis is most commonly caused by hypertrophy of the pyloric muscle, a condition known as congenital pyloric stenosis, in which the main symptom of PROJECTILE VOMITING often occurs 6 to 8 weeks after birth.

Suppuration

The process by which pus is formed during the course of an acute INFLAMMATION. Pus consists of dead and living polymorphonuclear leucocytes, other inflammatory cells and tissue cells which have been killed by microorganisms or other agents. The dead polymorphonuclear cells liberate digestive enzymes which cause liquefaction of the dead tissue cells. When the inflammatory reaction has been produced by bacteria the pus has a characteristic appearance according to the organism which is involved. Pus covering the surfaces of a burn which is infected with the bacterium known as *Pseudomonas aeruginosa* (pyocyaneus) has a characteristic greenish colour. Pus caused by a pyogenic (pus-forming) organism such as *Staphylococcus aureus*, responsible for boils and wound infections, is normally yellowish in colour.

Swelling, abdominal see ABDOMINAL SWELLING

Syncope see FAINTING

Tachycardia

An increase in the heart rate above the normal 70 to 80 beats/minute.

The rate of the normal heart is controlled by the sino-atrial node or 'pacemaker' from which 'impulses' arise which pass first through the atrial muscle to the atrio-ventricular node and then onwards down the bundle of His and throughout the muscle of the ventricles. Such impulses cause the rhythmic contration of the cardiac muscle which is the 'heart beat'. The rate of discharge of impulses from the sino-atrial node is, itself, controlled by the autonomic nervous system. Impulses from the vagus nerve normally inhibit the rate of discharge of the S-A node, whereas the sympathetic nerves excite the node and cause an increase in the number of impulses generated. Under normal circumstances the influence of the vagus nerve is the greater, with the result that the normal heart rate is slow. Should the vagal nerve fibres to the sino-atrial node be cut, the heart rate increases immediately.

Tachycardia can occur in a perfectly normal, healthy individual due to the following causes:

(1) Exercise. Tachycardia occurs because the muscles require an increased amount of blood, firstly to supply the oxygen necessary for the increased muscular activity and secondly to remove the products of tissue metabolism.

(2) Emotion. This causes an increase in the amount of adrenaline in the circulation which, in turn, produces an effect similar to stimulation of the sympathetic nerves.

(3) The excessive consumption of tobacco or alcohol, see PAROXYSMAL TACHYCARDIA

Tachycardia is a sign of certain pathological conditions:

(1) In any diseases causing FEVER the cardiac rate increases because of the increase in metabolism. Similarly tachycardia occurs in thyrotoxicosis.

181

(2) Following haemorrhage the heart rate increases in order to maintain the oxygen supply to the tissues with the reduced volume of blood in the circulation.

(3) In ANAEMIA, because the total oxygen-carrying capacity of the blood is reduced.

Tenesmus

A symptom consisting of straining in a desire to empty the lower bowel without defaecation taking place.

It occurs in the presence of any severe inflammatory lesion involving the lower rectum, such as proctocolitis or a specific dysentery. It is also common in the presence of polyp or carcinoma of the rectum when the tumour forms a 'pseudo-stool' which gives rise to the sensations necessary to excite defaecation.

Tetanus

A sign of infection by the anaerobic bacillus, *Clostridium tetani*, which causes its effect by the liberation of an exotoxin which passes from the site of infection via the motor nerves to affect the cells of the spinal cord.

The organism enters the tissues by a wound, and because it is anaerobic it will only proliferate in certain circumstances, i.e. when the wound is dirty, deep, contaminated and the blood supply to the tissues has been damaged. Once the toxin has reached the spinal cord it interferes with the control of the motor activity of the voluntary muscles in such a way that intermittent or continuous contraction of the affected muscle groups begins. When the contractions are continuous, an overall increase in tone occurs, whereas intermittent contraction causes muscular spasms with complete relaxation in between.

The involvement of only a few segments of the spinal cord causes local tetanus, but when greater quantities of exotoxin are formed and liberated, generalized CONVULSIONS and OPISTHOTONOS develop with death in a severe case usually caused by respiratory failure.

Involvement of the facial muscles causes a characteristic facial appearance known as the 'RISUS SARDONICUS'. Contraction of the muscles closing the jaw causes TRISMUS, a sign giving the condition its old name of lockjaw.

Tetany

A symptom associated with a low plasma calcium level, CARPO-PEDAL SPASM and a positive CHVOSTEK'S SIGN.

The cause of tetany is hyperexcitability of the junctional zone between the motor nerve ending and the muscle which is caused by the low plasma calcium. Common causes are:
   (1) Persistent feeding of a neonate on cow's milk.
   (2) Removal of the parathyroid glands during the operation of thyroidectomy.
   (3) ALKALOSIS caused by severe VOMITING, the excessive administration of alkalies or overbreathing.

Thrombocytopenia

A sign of a variety of conditions all of which lead, due to the reduction in platelet numbers, to extensive bruising and HAE-MATOMA formation even following slight injuries.

Thrombocytopenia has two main causes:
   (1) Failure of platelet production which may result from the destruction of the bone marrow by drugs or irradiation, replacement of the bone marrow by metastatic cancer or lastly from causes unknown.
   (2) Failure of platelet survival in the peripheral circulation which may result from unknown causes as in idiopathic thrombocytopenic PURPURA, drug sensitivity, infections, autoimmune reactions and excessive destruction of the platelets by the spleen, a condition known as hypersplenism.

Tic

A particular movement which is often repeated. Such movements are frequently manifestations of ANXIETY and may be little more than personal oddities.

The term is also used in describing the syndrome of trigeminal neuralgia, otherwise known as *'tic douloureux'* in which severe pain in the head and face occur together with repeated spasms of the facial muscles.

Tinnitus

Variously described by the sufferer as ringing, buzzing, hissing or singing in the ear, tinnitus is a relatively common symptom. It may precede conductive DEAFNESS when noises in or around the ear, which are normally masked by the hearing of outside noises may intrude on the patient's mind.

Tinnitus is also common in:

(1) Ménière's disease in which the labyrinth of the inner ear is grossly abnormal.
(2) Following high doses of certain drugs such as aspirin or quinine.
(3) Ischaemia of the auditory apparatus produced by anaemia or atheroma.

Tophi

Nodules found over the knuckles and pinna of the ear formed by the deposition of urate crystals in the subcutaneous tissues.

Such nodules are most commonly a sign of gout although they can occur in disease conditions associated with the excessive destruction of cells such as leukaemia or polycythaemia. Gout itself is an inherited defect in uric acid metabolism resulting in a high circulating level of uric acid. In addition to the characteristic tophi, the deposition of uric acid in joint tissues, particularly of the first metatarsal, leads to a gouty arthritis accompanied by severe attacks of pain, swelling and redness of the joint.

Torticollis

Otherwise known as wry neck, in which the neck is twisted to one side due to contraction of the sternomastoid muscle. The result is rotation of the face to the side opposite the contracting lesion together with flexion of the head to the contracted side.

Torticollis may be acute when it is usually a symptom and sign of prolapse of a cervical disc, inflamed cervical glands or less commonly, injury or actual disease of the cervical spine. Occasionally the torticollis is spasmodic, when it is usually a sign of some psychological disorder.

In the past congenital torticollis was not uncommon, the

usual cause being a sternomastoid tumour. This condition occurs following difficult labour or breech delivery, and is believed to be caused by the development of a venous thrombosis in the affected sternomastoid muscle. In nearly all such infants, a hard lump is noted in the sternomastoid on the affected side and as the swelling disappears, so the deformity develops. Left untreated, facial hemiatrophy occurs on the affected side. Very rarely congenital torticollis was due to congenital abnormality of the cervical vertebra.

Tremor

A tremor is a rhythmical movement at a joint brought about by alternating contractions of antagonistic groups of muscles.

A tremor may occur in a FUNCTIONAL condition such as HYSTERIA or ANXIETY, or it may be a sign of either a systemic illness or a specific disorder of the central nervous system. Systemic disorders associated with tremor include HYPERTHYROIDISM, alcoholism, HEPATIC FAILURE, respiratory failure and renal failure.

Disorders of the central nervous system may involve either the cerebral cortex, the basal ganglia or the cerebellum:

(1) Lesions of the cerebral cortex associated with tremor are nearly always accompanied by mental change, examples of this are general paralysis of the insane, caused by syphilitic INFLAMMATION of the brain, or by mercury poisoning.
(2) Lesions of the basal ganglia lead to the coarse slow tremor characteristic of PARKINSONISM.
(3) Lesions of the cerebellum or its communications lead to a type of tremor which is exaggerated by voluntary effort and is, therefore, known as an 'intention tremor'. This type of tremor can be demonstrated by asking the patient to touch the tip of his nose accurately with the tip of the index finger when the tremor is seen to become rapidly worse as the finger approaches the nose. Diseases affecting the cerebellum include multiple sclerosis, Friedreich's ataxia, neoplasms, vascular conditions and occasionally inflammatory conditions.

Trismus

Spasm of the jaw muscles, usually associated with severe TETANUS, hence the alternative name of lockjaw for this desease. Other causes include severe TETANY and rarely strychnine poisoning.

Trousseau's sign

CARPOPEDAL SPASM is evoked by squeezing the arm in patients suffering from latent tetany due to hyperexcitability of the neuromuscular junctions caused by a sudden reduction in the circulating calcium level. This can occur after parathyroidectomy for tumour or it can occur after the accidental removal of the parathyroid glands during thyroidectomy.

Turner's syndrome

A genetic condition associated with the presence of only one female (X) and no male (Y) chromosome. This genetic abnormality causes stunted growth, webbing of the neck and failure of testicular development, gonadal agenesis.

Ulceration

An ulcer is a break in the continuity of an epithelial surface. Ulceration is occasionally a sign of some systemic illness, for example, in congenital spherocytosis which is an uncommon cause of haemolytic ANAEMIA, ulceration of the legs may occur and in HYPERTENSION, widespread ulceration of the lower limbs is sometimes found (Martorelli's syndrome).

More commonly, however, ulceration is a sign of local disease in the affected tissues and the result of:

(1) Injury, as in dental ulcers which usually occur between the lip and gums caused by the pressure of ill-fitting dentures.

(2) Pyogenic infection. Acute inflammation involving a mucosal surface causes ulceration as in ulcerative colitis.

(3) Trophic ulceration. Adequate nutrition of the tissues depends upon an adequate blood supply and a properly functioning nerve supply. If either of these is inadequate,

ulceration follows. Therefore trophic ulceration is common in:

(a) Occlusive vascular disease caused either by arterial spasm or atherosclerosis due to inadequate nutrition.

(b) Certain conditions involving the peripheral nervous system such as diabetes mellitus, syphilis, peripheral neuropathy and peripheral nerve injury. In this group the ulcers commonly form on the sole of the foot and are of such depth that they are referred to as penetrating ulcers.

(4) Venous ulceration. A common cause of ulceration of the lower limb caused by inadequacy of the venous drainage of the affected limb.

(5) Specific infections such as:

(a) Syphilis. The ulcer of early syphilis is known as the primary chancre, and that of late syphilis, a gumma.

(b) Tuberculosis.

(c) Parasitic. *Leishmania tropica* can cause ulcers, usually about the face.

(6) Malignant disease. Ulcers due to malignant disease may affect any epithelial surface. Two special types of malignant ulceration are:

(a) The rodent ulcer which occurs on the face causing severe local destruction if untreated. This type of malignancy is unusual in that it does not cause metastases.

(b) The Marjolin's ulcer. This is a rare type of malignant ulcer occurring in an area of skin which has been the site of chronic irritation caused, for example, by burns or irradiation.

(7) Bed sore, decubitus ulcer.

Uraemia

A clinical syndrome produced by the biochemical abnormalities associated with acute or chronic renal failure. Whilst numerous biochemical changes have been identified in uraemia the exact interpretation of many of these remains to be established. The syndrome gained its name from the associated rise in the blood urea which is a constant feature of both acute and chronic renal failure although it is extremely doubtful whether this particular chemical substance is actually responsible for any of the metabolic changes or clinical features of the condition.

In both acute and chronic renal failure the following biochemical abnormalities develop:

(1) Disturbances of salt, potassium, calcium, magnesium and phosphate metabolism.

(2) An elevation of the blood urea which may rise rapidly or slowly depending upon the underlying condition and the rate at which this chemical compound is being produced.

(3) ACIDOSIS.

In addition the following clinical features occur:

(1) ANOREXIA, nausea and VOMITING.

(2) Intellectual deterioration followed by FITS.

(3) Furring of the tongue.

In chronic renal disease PROTEINURIA and CASTS are found and a characteristic pigmentation of the skin occurs which is usually associated with slight swelling of the eyelids.

In advanced renal failure CARDIAC ARREST may follow the elevated serum potassium, PURPURA may be associated with alteration of platelet function and severe convulsions may occur.

Acute renal failure is normally defined as a condition in which the output of urine suddenly falls below 400 ml/day. It may be a sign of:

(1) SHOCK (pre-renal failure) which may cause either a temporary renal disturbance or if prolonged, lead to structural changes known as renal tubular necrosis or cortical necrosis.

(2) Diseases of the kidney itself such as acute nephritis or the vascular changes of malignant HYPERTENSION.

(3) Obstruction to the normal outflow of urine from the kidney (post-renal), e.g. obstruction by stone of the ureter of a solitary kidney.

Chronic renal failure is a sign of a large variety of different conditions all of which affect the kidney including:

(1) Destructive diseases such as glomerulonephritis and polyarteritis nodosa.
(2) Infections such as pyelonephritis and tuberculosis.
(3) Obstruction to the urinary tract caused by prostatic obstruction.
(4) Congenital renal anomalies such as polycystic disease.
(5) HYPERTENSION.
(6) A variety of rarer conditions including gout, diabetes and myelomatosis.

Ureteric colic

An intermittent pain radiating from loin to groin which is a symptom associated with acute obstruction of the upper urinary tract, that is the kidney or ureter.

Commonly caused by the passage of a stone, it may occasionally result from blood clots. The colic is caused by the distension of the ureter proximal to the obstructing agent and to the excessive peristalsis which this causes. Should the stone impact at the junction of the ureter with the bladder, the patient often suffers from STRANGURY in addition to colic.

Urticaria

An acute or chronic disorder of the skin in which intensely itchy, white, elevated lesions surrounded by an erythematous halo develop. These lesions, known as weals, may last from a few minutes to several hours and then disappear without trace.

Urticaria is a sign of local ANAPHYLAXIS in which the reaction between antibody and antigen leads to the release of the chemical substance histamine, which causes capillary dilatation and an increase in its permeability. Acute urticaria is commonly caused by foods such as sea-food, eggs, milk and chocolates, by trauma or by drugs and it often begins with explosive suddenness and then gradually improves over a period of 7 to 10 days. The urticaria precipitated by drugs such as penicillin differs in that it may persist long after the drug has been withdrawn.

189

Vaginal discharge

A slight discharge is normally seen at the vulva. The discharge is a mixture of secretions arising from the Bartholin's, sebaceous and apocrine glands of the vulva and from the vaginal walls themselves, mainly due to the breakdown of desquamated epithelial cells lining the vagina, together with cervical mucus, the amount of which varies with the various phases of the menstrual cycle. Such normal secretions are increased in amount around the time of ovulation, a few days premenstrually, during pregnancy and during sexual arousal.

If excessive quantities of normal secretions occur, the term 'leucorrhoea' is used and this excess is mainly derived from the cervical component. It forms a brownish-yellow stain on the underclothes, often leading to the mistaken belief that the discharge contains blood.

An abnormal vaginal discharge is produced by:

(1) Infection involving:
   (a) The vulva and vagina by the gonococcus, *Trichomonas vaginalis* and *Candida albicans*.
   (b) The cervix, by the gonococcus or by secondary infection of an erosion.
   (c) The endometrium, by puerperal infection or tuberculosis.
(2) Neoplasms. Neoplasms exposed to the lumen of the genital tract cause increasing discharge. Should the neoplasm ulcerate the discharge becomes offensive, purulent and blood stained.
(3) Fistula formation:
   (a) Between the vagina and rectum, in which case a faecal discharge occurs.
   (b) Between the bladder and the vagina, causing persistent urinary incontinence.

Vertebro-basilar syndromes

Transient attacks of VERTIGO, hemiparesis, HEMIANOPIA, APHASIA, ATAXIA, sometimes accompanied by loss of memory, which are associated with partial occlusion of the vertebral and basilar arteries which supply the brain with blood.

Since the commonest cause of such occlusion is athero-sclerosis of the offending blood vessels, these attacks are more common after the age of 50. The same symptom complex also occurs in patients suffering from cervical spondylosis. In this condition bony spurs form on the cervical vertebrae and when the head is placed into a certain position, these bony promi-nences compress the vertebral artery as it passes through the vertebra. This results in a transient cerebral ischaemia.

Vertigo

Vertigo may be defined as a false sense of movement either of the patient himself (subjective vertigo) or of his surround-ings (objective vertigo). The sensation may be so extreme that an affected individual sways and falls to the ground. Pallor, sweating and VOMITING, denoting autonomic distress, commonly occur.

Vertigo is a symptom associated with a disturbance of one or more of the following:

(1) The vestibular apparatus in the inner ear.
(2) The vestibular division of the eighth cranial nerve.
(3) The vestibular nucleus in the brain stem.
(4) The connections of the vestibular nuclei in the brain stem to the cortex of the temporal lobes.
(5) The cerebellum.

When the vertigo arises from conditions outside the brain it is often termed peripheral, in contrast to central vertigo caused by lesions within the brain.

A common cause of peripheral vertigo is Ménière's disease, the cause of which is uncertain. This type of vertigo is usually paroxysmal and associated with DEAFNESS and often TINNITUS due to damage to the cochlear nerve. Other causes of peripheral vertigo include INFLAMMATION of the inner ear, injury causing HAEMORRHAGE and tumours. It can also be produced by irrigat-ing the external auditory meatus with cold water. This will cause vertigo and NYSTAGMUS and by comparing the onset of nystagmus in both eyes, the condition of the semicircular canals in the inner ear can be determined.

Central vertigo is usually due to arterial insufficiency caused by atheroma affecting the blood vessels supplying the cerebellum, multiple sclerosis or tumours particularly of the cerebellopontine angle.

Virilism

The gradual development of male secondary sexual characteristics in the female in which increasing hirsutism, deepening of the voice, acne, clitoral hypertrophy, thinning of the scalp hair and menstrual irregularity terminating in AMENORRHOEA occur.

Virilism may be:

(1) Idiopathic: Mild and even severe degrees of HIRSUTISM associated with other features of virilism may occur without any demonstrable endocrine abnormality other than an increased blood level of the androgenic steroids.

(2) A symptom of endocrine disorders particularly:

    (a) CUSHING'S SYNDROME. This is particularly so when the cushingoid appearance is due to a cancer of the adrenal gland.

    (b) A virilizing ovarian tumour which causes virilization by secreting the male hormone, testosterone.

    (c) Congenital adrenal hyperplasia which occurs in adolescent girls.

Visible peristalsis

The ability to see the peristaltic waves of the gastrointestinal tract depends upon the thickness of the abdominal wall.

If this is thin, as in the ageing multiparous female, the presence of visible peristalsis is of no significance. If, however, the abdominal wall is of normal thickness, distension together with visible peristalsis usually indicates the presence of intestinal obstruction. The precise pattern of the peristaltic waves gives some indication of the site of obstruction. Thus waves travelling across the upper abdomen from left to right indicate obstruction at the pylorus, whereas waves travelling in the opposite direction indicate a large bowel obstruction distal to the splenic flexure. When the small bowel is obstructed, as for example by an external hernia, the peristaltic waves form a 'ladder pattern' down the centre of the abdomen.

Vomiting

The forceful expulsion of gastric and intestinal contents through the mouth. This act is frequently preceded by TACHYCARDIA, salivation, sweating and pallor.

Vomiting begins with a deep inspiration, after which the glottis and the nasopharynx are closed to protect the air passages. A strong expiratory effort then occurs accompanied by a simultaneous contraction of the abdominal muscles. The increased intrathoracic and intra-abdominal pressure is transmitted to the stomach. At the same time both the upper part of the stomach and oesophagus relax whilst strong peristaltic waves sweep over the stomach from the pylorus to the body, expelling its contents into the oesophagus. The latter empties because of the raised intrathoracic pressure and some reversed peristalsis. Finally, breathing begins once again.

Vomiting is controlled by a vomiting centre in the brain stem. This can be stimulated directly by mechanical stimuli such as conditions causing a raised intracranial pressure, by chemical substances such as digitalis and apomorphine and by nervous REFLEXES originating in:

(1) The stomach and small intestine if these are distended as a result of mechanical obstruction.
(2) The cerebrum. Unpleasant sights, smells or events may cause vomiting.
(3) The inner ear. Disturbances of the inner ear are particularly liable to be associated with vomiting.

The character of the material vomited should always be noted since this may be of considerable diagnostic importance, for example a COFFEE-GROUND VOMIT indicates the presence of upper gastrointestinal haemorrhage.

See also PROJECTILE VOMITING.

Waardenburg's syndrome

A genetic condition transmitted by an autosomal dominant gene in which wide separation of the eyes occurs, together with deafness, and a white forelock. The eyes are also often different in colour.

Waterbrash

Occasionally occurring in a perfectly normal individual, waterbrash is the sudden filling of the mouth with saliva which of course has little if any taste, unlike regurgitated gastric juice which has a definite unpleasant taste. This symptom accompanies both oesophageal and gastric disorders and is probably caused by an exaggerated oesophago-salivary reflex.

Water-hammer pulse

Usually felt in the radial artery at the wrist, particularly when the arm is held vertically. The pulse beat strikes the palpating fingers suddenly and with great force, and just as suddenly becomes impalpable, hence the description.

This type of pulse is a sign that the aortic valves are incompetent and so permit aortic regurgitation to occur when ventricular contraction has ceased. The sign may, therefore, be present in any condition in which the aortic valves are damaged. Apart from congenital absence or deformity these conditions include 'rheumatic' heart disease, infective endocarditis and atherosclerotic heart disease.

In keeping with the physical characteristics of the pulse patients suffering from aortic regurgitation have an elevated systolic blood pressure, a decreased diastolic pressure and hence a very wide pulse pressure.

Waterhouse–Friderichsen syndrome

The development of profound SHOCK due to destruction of the adrenal glands in the course of a severe meningococcal SEPTICAEMIA. The glands are destroyed by sudden HAEMORRHAGE into their substance. This is caused by the sudden disruption of the capillary endothelium by the circulating toxin produced by the meningococcus which in addition also causes a profound reduction in the number of platelets in the circulation, thus increasing the haemorrhagic tendency. The shock occurring in this syndrome cannot be relieved without the administration of large doses of corticosteroids.

Weber's test

A test used to distinguish between conductive and perceptive DEAFNESS. The base of a vibrating tuning fork is applied to the top of the head in the midline. The sound is transmitted equally in a normal individual to the inner ear on both sides of the skull, but in a patient suffering from perceptive deafness the vibration is heard loudest in the ear with the better function. In conductive deafness the sound is transmitted to the ear with the greater conductive loss.

Wheeze

A sign of narrowing of the air passages. Wheezing is usually loudest during expiration because during this phase of respiration the air passages are narrowest due to a combination of their own elasticity and the gradually increasing intrathoracic pressure. Thus any narrowing already present is exaggerated.

The common conditions in which a wheeze may be heard include:

(1) Blockage of the air passages by mucus or a foreign body.
(2) Organic disease of the wall of the bronchi, either by INFLAMMATION or new growth.
(3) Spasm of the air passages due to abnormal muscular contraction as in asthma.

Whitlow

A sign of INFLAMMATION around the base of the nail, otherwise known as a paronychia. Most commonly the result of a staphylococcal infection but occasionally due to a fungus infection and rarely the virus causing herpes.

Winged scapula

A sign of wasting or PARALYSIS of the muscle known as the serratus anterior which holds the scapula in apposition to the chest wall. This muscle is supplied by the long thoracic nerve which may be injured during the performance of a radial mastectomy. The scapula may appear to be in a normal position, but if the affected individual is asked to raise the arms to 90 degrees and to push against a wall, the backward projection of the vertebral border of the scapula (winging) becomes obvious. The disability produced by such a lesion is minimal.

Wrist-drop

A sign of injury to or disease of the radial nerve in which the person is unable to dorsiflex the wrist and extend the digits. Because the radial nerve is primarily a motor nerve, the anaesthesia resulting from the damage is usually confined to a small area on the back of the thumb and the skin between this and the index finger.

Xanthelasma

The subcutaneous deposition of fat and cholesterol in the eyelids leading to yellowish raised patches. Such patches may be associated with an abnormally high level of cholesterol in the blood and the development of premature atherosclerosis of the arteries with the attendant possibilities of a STROKE or cardiac infarct.

Zollinger–Ellison syndrome

Severe and intractable duodenal ULCERATION, often associated with a severe watery DIARRHOEA. The basic cause is a tumour of the islets of Langerhans in the pancreas. This tumour secretes excessive amounts of the hormone known as gastrin which is a powerful stimulator of gastric secretion. In the presence of gastrin over-secretion the stomach produces excessive quantities of acid and pepsin which lead to mucosal ulceration and an acid-induced enteritis which causes the DIARRHOEA.